HEALTH SYSTEMS RESEARCH

Edited by K. Davis and W. van Eimeren

Indicators and Trends in Health and Health Care

Edited by Detlef Schwefel

With 7 Figures

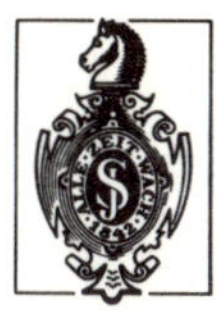

Springer-Verlag Berlin Heidelberg New York
London Paris Tokyo

Professor Dr. rer. pol. Detlef Schwefel
Gesellschaft für Strahlen- und
Umweltforschung mbH München
MEDIS – Institut für Medizinische
Informatik und Systemforschung
Ingolstädter Landstraße 1
D-8042 Neuherberg

ISBN 3-540-16998-9 Springer-Verlag Berlin Heidelberg New York
ISBN 0-387-16998-9 Springer-Verlag New York Berlin Heidelberg

Library of Congress Cataloging-in-Publication Data
Indicators and trends in health and health care.
(Health systems research)
1. Health status indicators–Congresses.
2. Medical care–Forecasting–Congresses.
3. Public health–Forecasting–Congresses.
I. Schwefel, Detlef. II. Series. [DNLM: 1. Delivery of Health Care–trends. 2. Health Services Research.
3. Health Status Indicators. 4. Health Surveys. W 84.1 I39]
RA407.A2I53 1987 362.1 86-26294
ISBN 0-387-16998-9 (U.S.)

Printed in Germany

Printing and Bookbinding: Druckhaus Beltz, 6944 Hemsbach/Bergstraße
2119/3145-543210

Table of Contents

List of Contributors

Dr. Jean-Pierre Bendel
Brookdale Institute of Gerontology
POB 13087
Jerusalem 91130
Israel

Dott. Lamberto Briziarelli &
Dott.ssa. Nerina Dirindin
CRESA
C.so Massimo d'Azeglio 42
I-10125 Torino
Italy

Karen Davis, Ph.D.
Professor & Chairman
Department of Health Policy and Management
School of Hygiene and Public Health
Johns Hopkins University
624 N. Broadway
Baltimore, MD 21205
USA

Mårten Lagergren, Ph.D.
Forskningsrådsnämnden
Secretariat for Futures Studies
Box 6710
S-113 85 Stockholm
Sweden

Prof. Manfred A. Max-Neef
Director
CEPAUR (Development Alternatives Centre)
Casilla 27 095
Santiago 27
Chile

Jerrold S. Maxmen, M.D.
Associate Professor of Clinical Psychiatry
Columbia University
College of Physicians & Surgeons
New York City
USA

Prof. Alexander Petrovski
Institute for Control Science of the Academy of Sciences
Profsoyuznaya 65
Moscow 117 342
USSR

Jean-Pierre Poullier
Directorate for Social Affairs, Manpower & Education
OECD
2 rue André Pascal
F-75775 Paris Cedex 16
France

Uwe E. Reinhardt, Ph.D.
James Madison Professor of Political Economy
Princeton University
Princeton, New Jersey
USA

Elisabeth Schach, Dipl.Volkswirt
Universität Dortmund
Hochschulrechenzentrum
Bittermarkstraße 96
Postfach 50 05 00
D-4600 Dortmund 50
FRGermany

Prof. Dr. Detlef Schwefel
MEDIS-Institut der GSF
Ingolstädter Landstraße 1
D-8042 Neuherberg
FRGermany

Gail R. Wilensky, Ph. D. &
Steven Chapman
Project HOPE
Health Sience Education Center
Millwood, Virginia 22646
USA

Indicators and Trends in Health and Health Care
- Introduction -

Detlef Schwefel

Scope and Purpose

The papers contained in this book originate from two conferences, held in Munich on July 19, 1984, whose subjects were "Indicator-Based Reporting Systems" and "Long-Term Trend Indicators and Models". These conferences were autonomous parts of the "Third International Conference on System Science in Health Care"; they were organized by the MEDIS Institute of Medical Informatics and Health Services Research of the GSF Research Centre, and were sponsored by the German Federal Ministry of Research and Technology. Their purpose was to discuss the priority and relevance of, and to prepare terms of reference for, research to be undertaken and promoted in the Federal Republic of Germany on trends and indicators of health and health care. It is believed, though, that the revised papers (the last was received end of 1985) which make up this book may be of interest for a wider audience.

Research Programme

In 1978, the West German government launched a Research Promotion Programme for Health and Health Care. This programme, revised in 1983, aims at building up and strengthening research capacities, not only in the traditional domains of clinical research, but also for health services research, i.e. for research on the processes, structures and outcomes of health care, as well as on the planning of the care system. In planning, special attention should be given to two areas of research:

1. Indicator-based reporting systems for health and health care
2. Long-term trends in health and health care

Indicator Systems

By the topic "Indicator-based reporting systems for health and health care", the three federal ministries responsible, i.e. the Ministry of Research and Technology, the Ministry of Labour and Social Affairs, and the Ministry of Youth, Family and Health[1] understand the following:

> Studies are to be promoted that aim at relating the resources of the health care system to the most serious health risks, the most wide-spread illnesses, and the services performed and outcomes achieved in combating them. Through these projects the introduction of a regular reporting system for health is to be made possible. The plan of an indicator-based reporting system for health, as developed during the previous programme period, is to be gradually completed and to be tested in practice. The possibilities inherent in the data available, especially the information contained in the routine data of the Statutory Health Insurance, should be used more widely. In addition, new instruments are to be developed in order to fill information gaps, particularly with respect to objectively existing and subjectively felt health risks as well as to the morbidity of the population. Use should be made of the instrument of "health surveys", as it is known in Anglo-Saxon countries; in doing so, attention should be paid to the possible linking of data on risks and morbidity with data on the services, structures and financing of the health system so that comprehensive accounts can be achieved.

Long-Term Trends

The governmental research programme regarding "Long-term trends in health and health care"[2] reads as follows:

> The nationally and internationally existing options for the long-term development of the health care system are to be examined more intensively. Special attention will be paid to the importance of secular trends (demographic development; of changes in health risks, in the spectrum of diseases, and in medical technology); and of alternative health care structures for the improvement of the health status of the population. Experiences from foreign care systems, which in spite of their different structures are confronted with largely similar problems, are to be scientifically examined, assessed and presented to the public discussion in the Federal Republic of Germany. For this purpose, a scientific basis has to be laid for a health policy that starts from vital health-related problems and needs rather than focusing on the institutional conditions of the health care system or some organizational and financial questions. The research started during the previous programme, on the basis of model simulation and scenario techniques, is to be intensified and supplemented by internationally comparable studies on the essential structure variables of the health care system. These studies will, at the same time, contribute to the programme of the World Health Organization for the year 2000 and to the third research programme of the European Community, adopted in 1982, for medicine and health care.

---

1 Der Bundesminister für Forschung und Technologie, Der Bundesminister für Arbeit und Sozialordnung, Der Bundesminister für Jugend, Familie und Gesundheit (eds) (1983) *Forschung und Entwicklung im Dienste der Gesundheit. Programm der Bundesregierung* 1983-1986. Bonn, p 56

2 Ibid., pp 55-56

Tasks and Selection

The ministries are now preparing a national call for tenders in these areas of research. Our meeting was, at least implicitly, intended to formulate some terms of reference for studies on indicator systems and on long-term trends in health care. As the presentations and discussions were to stimulate German health services research, contributors were invited from several countries to report on their national and international experiences. Several sessions of the Third International Conference on System Science in Health Care[3] dealt with indicators, and some papers with trends. There were sessions on "Health System Performance Indicators", "Health Status Indicators" and "Health Information System Design"; in addition, a WHO Workshop on "Information Systems and Indicators for Strategies for HFA 2000" and another on "Information Needs of Primary Health Care" were held. The speakers in all these sessions had been asked to join the special one-day conference on trends and indicators in order to present their points of view during the discussion, i.e. to complement the invited papers, which, by the way, cannot be regarded as representative of the field under study. A third group of especially invited guests – well-known scientists in health services research from West Germany – had the opportunity of bringing in their questions and arguments, thus widening the discussion on indicators and trends. All these participants were asked to contribute short papers; a few did so.

Indicator Session

When we speak of indicator(-based reporting) systems, it is not only a matter of preparing one national report on health and health care. Rather, we consider a system of direct and indirect information from different sources – routine data, survey data, official data, etc. – about processes, structures and outcomes of the health care system, an indicator system which should be useful for decision support, activity reinforcement, planning, evaluation, monitoring and surveillance, and be flexible enough to be used at different regional, functional or organizational levels of different sectors or subsectors of health care systems. Such an indicator system can rely on modern technology, especially the tools of modern informatics; it should be comprehensive as well as comprehensible, and be permanently updated; it should also be cost-effective (which may mean that, for some problems, small scale surveys could be more adequate than the handling of large data files). Of course, research reality is, and probably will remain, far behind the ideals mentioned; but, as challenges, they will stimulate efforts. The invited papers for this special session deal with some selected but decisive aspects:

1. The first paper, given by Lamberto Briziarelli and Nerina Dirindin, deals with a case study in the region of Piedmont in Italy and presents an indicator system for the economic evaluation of health plan strategies

---

[3] Eimeren van, W., Engelbrecht, R. and Flagle, Ch. D. (eds): *Third International Conference on System Science in Health Care*. Springer-Verlag, Berlin Heidelberg New York Tokyo 1984

2. Jean-Pierre Bendel from Israel reports on his experiences in implementing an information system which considers the interests of its producers and its users alike
3. Jean-Pierre Poullier from France describes the experience the Organization for Economic Cooperation and Development (OECD) had when trying to stimulate and coordinate health indicator systems of different nations
4. Finally, Karen Davis from Baltimore focuses on indicator systems for future oriented analyses of health problems and, taking the example of the elderly, gives her ideas on the technology of presentation

After the presentation of these invited papers, a panel discussion took place where speakers from other sessions related with indicator systems as well as German experts discussed the topic intensively and extensively.

Trend Session

Long-term trends in health and health care may be seen from at least three different angles. First, a retrospective time series analysis could, for example, be used to identify trends, and interrelationships between trends, of economic development, health and their intervening factors alike. Second, by means of cross-sectional data, e.g. on differing development stages or different age structures, it might be possible to simulate variations in time or time series and to project them from the present into the future. Third, extrapolation, projection, imagination, even fantasy and day-dreaming may yield insights into alternative futures.

1. Gail Wilensky and Steven Chapman from the HOPE project explore demographic and other trends of the future
2. Elisabeth Schach comments on this paper
3. Alexander Petrovski from the USSR contributes a short statement on the theory of homogeneous populations
4. Uwe Reinhardt from Princeton argues on manpower projections; this area has been most prominent in long-term trend research
5. Jerrold S. Maxmen reconsiders his theses on the "post-physician era"
6. Besides these sectoral approaches to demography, manpower and knowledge, Mårten Lagergren reports on his programme to project welfare trends in Sweden from the past into the future
7. Lastly, Manfred A. Max-Neef from Chile, alternative Nobel prize winner of 1983, presents some reflections on the world-wide picture and international trends in health and health care

Conclusion

It is hoped that this quite heterogeneous discussion will stimulate health services research in various countries and settings, and that the approaches presented here will prove useful starting points.

Indicators of Health and Health Care

1. An Indicator System for the Evaluation of Public Health Programmes: The Case of the Region of Piedmont

Lamberto Briziarelli and Nerina Dirindin

The Italian public health sector was radically reformed in 1978. The new national health service replaced the previous system which was based on several uncoordinated and mostly single-purpose agencies. At present the National Health Service operates at three levels:

1. Central: the state level
2. Intermediate: the twenty-one regional governments
3. Local: the 671 so-called Unità Sanitarie Locali (USL) or local health units

Planning is essential for efficient management of limited resources and in order to achieve health reform targets at all three levels. The adoption of such planning methods encounters various problems, both theoretical and practical. For these reasons the central government in Italy has so far been unable to implement the new national health plan. Nevertheless some regional governments have enforced their own plans. Thus the Piedmont regional social health plan (RSHP) for the period 1982-1984 was adopted in 1982. It considers explicitly the problems of *evaluation* of the performance of the regional health services and of the fulfilment of the plan's objectives.

Evaluation must be based on *indicators*. That is why the regional government of Piedmont has entrusted various research centres with the construction of a *system of indicators*. A regional committee supervises both the building up and the testing of the system. The study was carried out by two working groups, each concentrating on one of the two basic aspects inherent in health service appraisal, namely:

1. Improvement in health and conditions of risk and damage (which we will call effectiveness)
2. Optimal use of employed resources (efficiency)

During the first stage of the study, the two working groups functioned autonomously, but met occasionally to share their findings and conclusions. They applied different, but compatible research approaches. Research into effectiveness particularly involved *problem areas* and *objectives*, while research into efficiency particularly involved the various departments or *services* projected in the USL.

The partition above is due to the way the project was developed. At first the Centro di Ricerca per l'Economia, l'Organizzazione e l'Amministrazione della Sanita (CRESA) was only asked to undertake that part of the study relating to efficiency. The work would in any case have had to be shared for operational reasons and the different areas of specialization required. Efficiency study is particularly directed towards topics of medical economy, whereas the effectiveness study centres on epidemiology. The setting up of two working groups reflected this need for professionalism while at the same time providing some overlap. The two groups have reached different stages in their analyses: the research into efficiency is almost completed while that into effectiveness is still under way. When both groups have reached the same stage, their results may be merged. The remainder of this paper is divided into two sections. The first, relating to research into efficiency, examines procedure, problems and results, while the second, relating to research into effectiveness, examines procedure and prospects for future development.

Table 1 summarizes health services components and relationships that can, in general, help build up a functional analysis of the National Health Service. It is obvious that the logical diagram shown in Table 1 may give rise to different sets of indications, depending on how one views the health service and its proposed objectives.

Efficiency Aspects

An Analytical Framework

Table 2 summarizes the indicators resulting from the study of health services efficiency. The object of the research into efficiency concerns only a part of the whole system of relationships shown in Table 1. The following families of indicators emerge:

1. Resources
2. Activities
3. Efficiency
4. Various (accessibility, vertical and horizontal integration, patient and personnel comfort, etc.)

The last group of indicators is explained by the need to match resources and activities with factors relating to service users (accessibility indicators) and inherent in the services themselves (comfort indicators), as well as by the need to follow an important aspect of the organization which also forms an intermediate objective in the regional plan (integration indicator). Territorial and population size (indicating number of potential users), to which resources and activities are related, are the only external system factors covered by the efficiency study.

After identifying the different indicator categories given above, it was also necessary to divide the whole system horizontally into individual, internally homogeneous sections; it was therefore divided into different operational fields or *services*. The following 10 services are envisaged by the regional health plan: public health, veterinary, legal medicine, primary health services, pharmaceutical services, primary integrative services, social assistance services, accounting and budgeting, general supplies and engineering, administration of personnel, property and legal

Table 1. Main national health service indicators

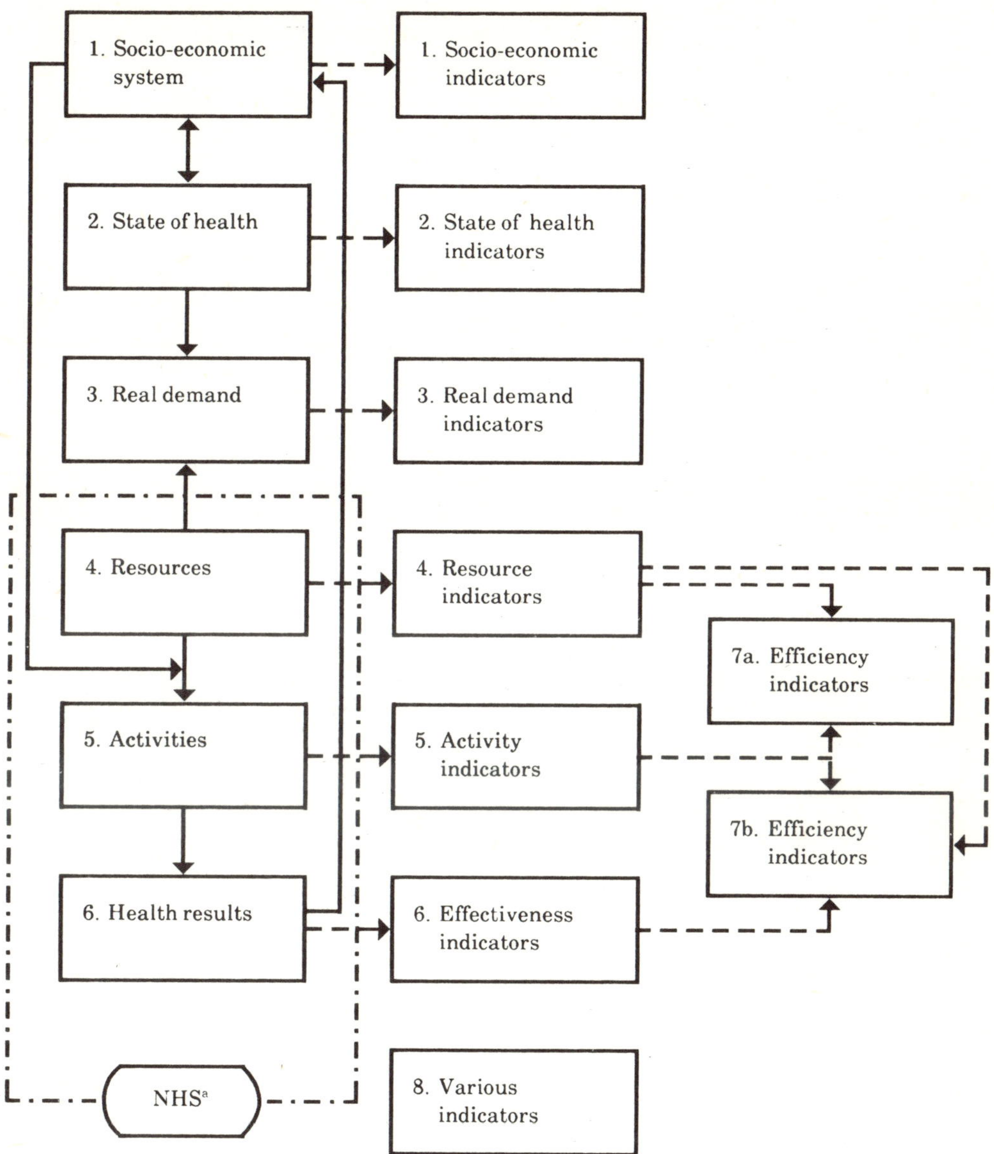

[a] National health service

matters. The different services are sometimes complementary and interchangeable, and this fact has not been ignored. Attention is paid, on the one hand, *to integration indicators*, and, on the other, to the efforts made in facing up to one of the most knotty problems encountered during the research: the identification of standard classification and measurement procedures to permit researchers to compare and combine services.

Table 2. Indicators used in the research into efficiency

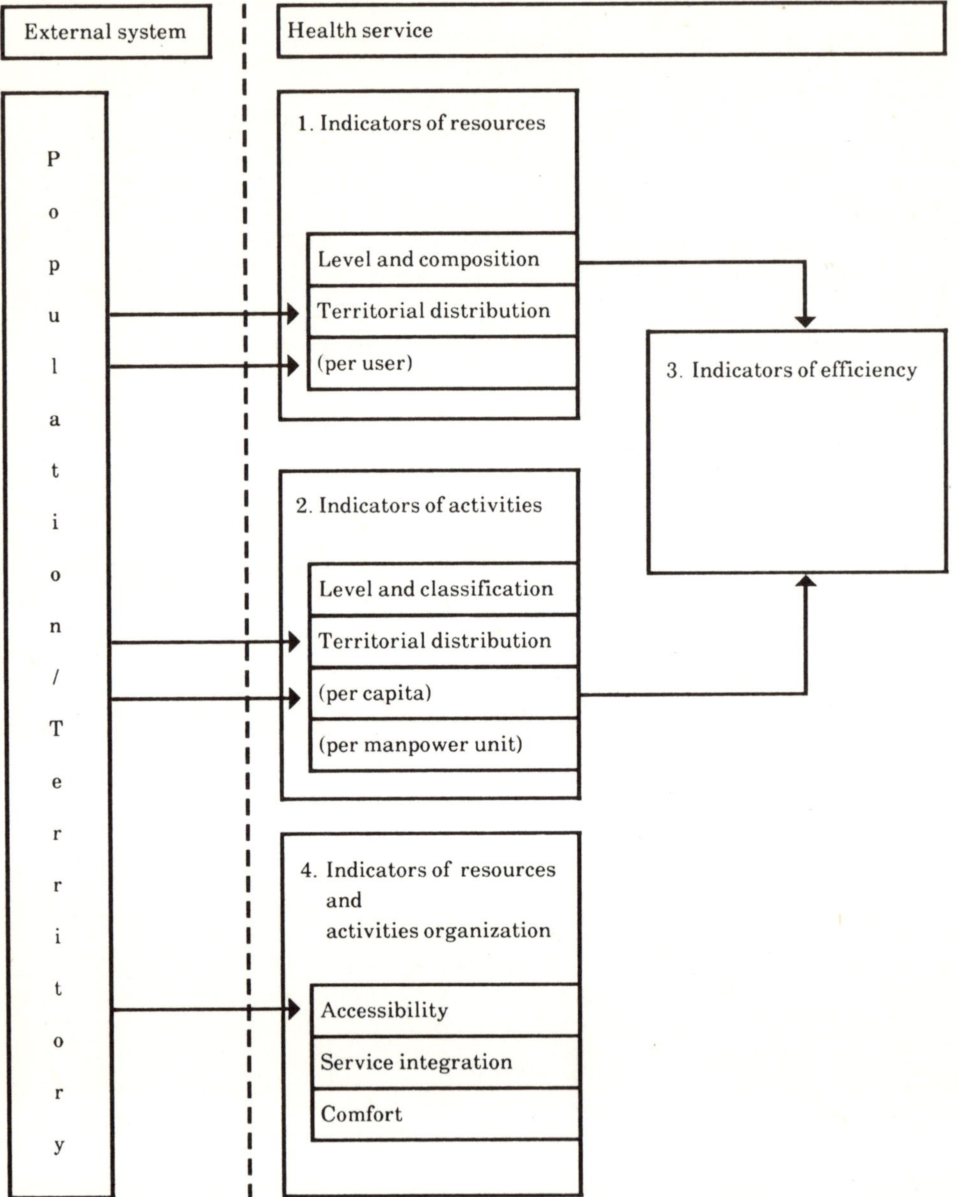

Table 3. Resources

Type of resources	Classification criteria	Calculation criteria	Weighting systems
Finances	Alternative classification criteria: - By purpose - By function - By cost centre - On the basis of financial stages Possible ranges: - Current revenues/expenses - Capital revenues/expenses	Monetary measurements (current prices)	
Personnel	Alternative classification criteria on the basis of: - Legal labour relationship - Functional labour relationship - Professional qualification	Theoretical physical units Real physical units Monetary measurements	Need for weighting systems based on contract characteristics (working hours, maximum rates for conventional activities)
Buildings	Alternative classification criteria on the basis of: - Dimension - Destination (functional areas)	Physical units Monetary measurements	No physical unit weighting system is envisaged, only similar immovables are added to one another
Movable property	Classification on the basis of asset nature They are divided up as follows: - Technical-health equipment - Accommodating equipment - Technical-economic equipment - Office furniture - Office equipment - Data processing equipment	Physical units Monetary measurements	No physical unit weighting system is envisaged, only similar movable assets important for their characteristic nature and/or economic relevance are added to one another (those belonging to the same category)
Consumables	Classification on the basis of asset nature with exclusive reference to assets important for their charcteristic nature and/or economic relevance	Physical units Monetary measurements	Need for weighting systems for additions within individual asset categories (pharmaceutical products in particular)

Definitions, Classifications, Units of Measurement and Weighting Systems

The first major task in the work schedule was the preparation of a progress report, called the *reference grid*, containing the definitions, classification criteria, calculation and weighting systems applied to the following data:

1. Resources, both financial and physical (personnel, buildings, movable property, consumables)
2. Activities
3. Accessibility

As there are no nationally or internationally accepted conventions in classification, we decided that it was necessary, as a first step, to set down the procedures by which factors indispensable to regional health service economic evaluation are identified and measured. This phase of the project was necessary for two reasons: (a) practical necessity (indicator system testing requires precise input data definition), and (b) clarification of theoretical-methodological questions (problems of basic data identification and measurement must be resolved before an indicator system can be constructed). The results of this work are summarized in Tables 3, 4 and 5. It should be emphasized that any choices made at this stage were closely determined by the objectives of the study.

Indicator Card and Base-Measurement Card

The working group then went on to prepare two card models: the base-measurement card and the indicator card.

From an operational viewpoint, the definition and implementation of an indicator system requires the preparation of a *set of indicator cards* (and, as a back-up, of *base-measurement cards*) that are concise and easy to consult. These cards would be available to sectorial operators for the purposes of information and critical appraisal. The practical application of this type of working tool became evident during the early stages of the study and was determined by the enormous quantity of material and the diverse nature of indicators marking meaning and content. The

Table 4. Activities

Classification of reference units	Calculation criteria	Need for weighting systems on the basis of
Population Users Cases treated Cases admitted Complex services Simple services Simple service elements	Physical units	Population factors Complexity of cases treated Service characteristics (simple or complex)

Table 5. Accessibility

Reference factors	Indicator categories
Location	Service location Architectural constraints
Socio-economic	Economic constraints
Organisation	Opening hours Booking procedure Service procedure Service integration
Cultural[a]	User education, information and participation
Psychological[a]	User satisfaction Service comfort Operator behaviour

[a] This kind of indicator is used to measure the effectiveness, too

main, significant features of each indicator, its possible interpretations, and its requirements were summarized on one single table: the indicator card. The base-measurement card, conversely, provides a statistical data back-up for the indicator card and contains all information relating to the technical-statistical properties of the various components considered necessary for indicator construction.

The *indicator card* model is shown in Table 6. This version may be revised in the light of efficiency and effectiveness study results. Although decisions to include or exclude certain problem areas or definitions when preparing the card may seem insignificant, they actually depend (directly or indirectly) on the initial premises laid down by the research group when defining their procedural approach.

Indicators Considered and Criteria for Choice

On the basis of the above reference grid, the subsequent stage is the identification of a large range of indicators to represent findings in the literature and research group suggestions. Selection made at this level only concerns the degree to which indicators relate to the object and purpose of the investigation and not to the availability or reliability of empirical data. This means that the list that we have called *indicators considered* is to be taken as pertinent and practically exhaustive, but not operational. A rigorous selection process is applied to this list to produce a condensed list of *proposed indicators* for research. This result is obtained by reducing both the number of factors examined and the number of associated indicators.

For the first criterion, wide use is made of two-stage analysis logic. According to this method, indicators should essentially highlight results that are ambiguous or

Table 6. Indicator card

Name	
Technical Description	
Definition of terms	
Phenomena to be checked	1 . . . . 2 . . . . 3 . . . .
Area of application	. . . . (USL function breakdown) . . . .
Plan reference	☐ Specific policies . . . . ☐ Objective projects . . . . ☐ Socially relevant actions . . . .
Class	☐ Resources ☐ Efficiency ☐ Integration ☐ Activity ☐ Accessibility ☐ Various
Relationship with other indicators	☐ Independent ☐ Complementary with . . . . ☐ Other connections . . . .
Space / time context	☐ Department . . . . ☐ Health centre . . . . ☐ Centre . . . . ☐ Health area . . . . ☐ District . . . . ☐ Region . . . . ☐ Commune . . . . ☐ . . . .
Statistical sources	☐ Autonomously obtainable at . . . . support . . . . Body responsible / How often / Operator Collection . . . . / . . . . / . . . . . . Processing . . . . / . . . . / . . . . . . Diffusion . . . . / . . . . / . . . . . . Reliability good ☐ adequate ☐ poor ☐
	☐ Obtainable by . . . .
	☐ Not autonomously obtainable
Value for assessment of RHSP	☐ Essential ☐ Useful ☐ . . . .
Notes	. . . .

Prerequisites:

Prerequisites \ Phenomena	1	2	3
Pertinence			
Specificity			
Precision			
Empirical aspects			
Overall judgement			

that do not tally with the regional plan. The task of checking, explaining and suggesting remedies is left to subsequent investigations. Sometimes similar procedures may be applied to consider the overall situation rather than its individual components (when it is reasonably safe to assume that components are not subject to opposing forces). At other times, the process may be simplified by identifying *sentinel events or guide services* to acceptably represent large groups of factors thanks to the presence of strong, stable internal correlations.

For the second selection criterion, cases where several indicators represent the same aspect of a phenomenon are systematically eliminated.

One more obvious selection criterion depends on the operational aspect, that is the availability and reliability of base data and collection and processing costs. The impact of this criterion may be minimized, on the one hand, by recommending collection of base measurements relating to indicators of particular interest only and, on the other, by trying to identify base measurements useful in the construction of more than one indicator.

Effectiveness Aspects

Methodology

Traditionally the measurement of effectiveness is based on the results of epidemiological surveys. These give some idea of the induced effect of health conditions, expressed in the negative terms of symptoms, diseases and handicaps.

Over the last few years, our ideas about health have undergone profound changes, as indeed have associated cultural reference points. This is manifest in the regulations underlying the new health services organization, which to a large extent supersede the traditional epidemiological survey method to make way for other factors, namely prevention (and not only the cure) of diseases, public participation, and the fact that all subjects using the health services do so on an equal footing. These new factors, incorporated in the Piedmont Regional Social Health Plan have, therefore, also been adopted as reference points for our study.

The underlying concept is the same as that already applied for efficiency indicators, except that selected indicators are not allocated according to services, but according to larger, more general target areas - the overall targets for these areas were clearly defined and several services and operators were responsible for different area functions. This allowed us to overcome the obstacle of the non-evaluability of, or the difficulty in evaluating, the effectiveness of an individual service or structure by including the action of each service in overall results obtained from the activity of coherent units of structures, departments and services. To do this, as a basic analysis unit we chose a minimum comprehensive unit of services, all having a common target that may be evaluated in terms of effectiveness. As the regional health service is still in its infancy, this analysis was limited to factors which may be unequivocally evaluated and constitute, at the same time, an extrememely significant operational framework connected to certain important regional social health plan targets.

The selected target areas are as follows: mother and child health care, health care for the elderly, health care for workers, prevention of disabilities and care for the disabled, environmental care, animal husbandry, emergency services.

Selected Indicators

Within the framework of the study, a limited number of indicators from different categories were selected in relation to their application within the social health plan to assess to what extent the operations carried out can improve the health of the population.

Effectiveness, in the strict sense of the word, is not evaluated, but rather the effective use of services and, consequently, the results that may be attributed to this set of factors. It should, however, be remembered that recorded changes are also linked to many other, more complex, social, economic or environmental factors. These factors justify the constant emphasis on the global nature of health matters and the fact that the importance of the determinant role of the health service cannot be overestimated. In this way the concept of efficacy expands to embrace a wider range of service characteristics. This more generalized concept covers other *service use indices of effectiveness*, such as accessibility and satisfaction indicators.

Up to this point our studies have been mainly centred on health result indicators, but they have been extended whenever possible to cover corresponding accessibility and quality indicators.

The outcome indicators we selected are of three types:

1. *Sentinel events* (corresponding to the formula *not cases of*...) only one of which is sufficient to trigger off an alarm
2. *Ratios or rates:* the tendency of these to modify over a given time scale is analysed
3. *Differential ratios or rates:* distributions are analysed in different population aggregations in relation to predicted distributions or to the mean regional population distribution. They are used to emphasize territorial, behavioural or other inequalities in service uses

Finally, we have used another type of indicator, *required existence* (presence/ absence), where the presence of a service or activity, even at a minimum level, is to be regarded as an important element.

A Standardized Indicator Classification Scheme

The construction of a standardized effectiveness indicator classification scheme has been attempted (which may subsequently be extended to efficiency indicators).

Distinct indicator groups were established in relation to the general and specific objectives of the health service as a whole. In this context, a system based on the aggregation of indicator sets standardized by net results is envisaged:

1. Behaviour indicators
2. Inequality indicators
3. Product indicators
4. Quality of life indicators

Behaviour Indicators

These observations allow us to evaluate the influences (negative and positive) that the health service as a whole exerts on the set of individuals and the extent to which the service determines positive attitudes and behaviours with respect to health matters. They include (a) parameters specifically applicable in the analysis of effects produced by strictly educational programmes (health education campaigns aimed at specific groups according to risk, territory, environment, physiological conditions, etc.), and (b) parameters necessary to emphasize the influence that health programmes and services (behaviour of operators, service procedures, departmental distribution network, type of services, homogeneity factors, equality, accessibility, etc.) generally exert on the population.

Knowledge of the above observations is necessary in order to measure real needs, avoid mechanisms of induced demand in the health sector and services in general, and prevent the introduction of further social control mechanisms through the health system.

Inequality Indicators

These indicators permit us to emphasize the level of democracy effectively achieved and practised within the framework of and through the health services and to what extent citizens are in a position to share equally in the benefits of the services available. This, in turn, gives us extremely useful guidelines for the integration of target projects, for dealing with cases of particular privation and also for the better gearing of service operation to the needs of users as a whole.

Some of the parameters to be pinpointed are directly derived from the population (connected to behaviour indicators or sometimes their derivatives) and others from an analysis of services and their operation. In the first stage of application of these evaluative techniques we can use service indicator results and consult observations deriving from service analyses for the part relating to the population.

Product Indicators

The product indicators generally comprise a group of already studied indicators, albeit only very approximate, partly applied in service analysis attempts. Under this general heading we may group some "effectiveness" and "efficiency" indicators. More generally, it may also cover so-called "cost indicators", i.e. the group of variables necessary to evaluate health service activities as a whole in strictly economic terms. It is preferable, however, to cover economic evaluation indicators in a separate sector to distinguish them from those necessary for the measurement of efficiency in the strict sense of the term.

It is possible to identify two groups of observations amongst the product indicators. One is directed at the study of the effects produced by the action on the set of factors making up the population's "state of health". The second is necessary for the analysis of quality and technical-scientific aspects of the service, in addition to the sheer quantity of services. Examples of observations are:

1. Risk factors, symptoms, disabilities, illnesses, death
2. Service quantity per service, per operator, per user, in relation to operational standards
3. Service quality, including
   - Errors in diagnosis - errors in treatment
   - Number or type of symptoms omitted when evaluating a disease
   - Combination of incompatible drugs
   - Hours spent waiting in outpatient departments and health centres
   - Days spent waiting for diagnoses, treatment, etc.
   - Difference between diagnosis on admission and diagnosis on discharge
   - Number of diagnostic tests per diagnosis

Quality of Life Indicators[1]

Quality of life indicators comprise a compound set of observable factors which should, when taken together, represent the general welfare of a population. These factors are not all precisely definable and definite, and naturally they take account of the historical and developmental stage that a given population has reached and also, therefore, of the subjective effect of this on the quality of life under the existing conditions. These observations may be divided into three different categories, dependent on economic, social and strictly health aspects.

Conclusions

As a result of the study described above, a list of indicators will be identified in order to evaluate the more important aspects of the national health service in Italy and the import of the first regional social health programme. The system will be completed soon. It will be tested in six local health units chosen to represent the whole regional health service.

---

1 A guideline of this type was also given by the World Health Organization in the context of its project on the adoption of appropriate lifestyles with the goal of "Health for all by 2000" in view.

At this stage of the research the following conclusions can be drawn:

1. In any program, the objectives to be attained must be clearly identified in the light of existing situations and available resources.
2. The major difficulty in improving the methods by which health programs are planned, controlled and evaluated is the lack of satisfactory measures of the end results of health care.
3. Further studies of the behaviour of professionals and users are necessary to check impact on needs, demand and results.
4. Manpower involvement and cooperation are necessary to achieve the evaluation of health programs in practice.
5. The system of indicators is one of many tools in evaluating health programs; its usefulness can be substantially increased by the simultaneous adoption of additional techniques of evaluation.
6. A large number of measures are essential for construction of a list of indicators that are sufficiently satisfactory and expressive.
7. In any case, the system of indicators can only point out abnormal positions; it cannot pass any judgement (negative or positive) on situations identified. It operates as an alarm clock; further studies may allow detailed evaluations.

2. Review of Computerized Information Systems in the Health Area and Their Implication for Long-Term Care

Jean-Pierre Bendel

The first observation that I made in reviewing health information systems (HISs) was a strong correlation between the level on which an HIS is used for policy making, planning or management, and its classification according to the three following groups:

1. The agency who controls the HIS is also the one who uses the information it generates and, furthermore, provides the input to it. Many institution-specific management information systems fall in this category.
2. The agency who controls the HIS also uses the information it generates, but has little control over the data input providers. This category includes, for example, cancer registries which are usually controlled by the same researchers as analyse them but who depend on the goodwill of hospitals, laboratories and others to provide the input data needed to create and update the registers.
3. The agency who controls the HIS has little contact with the potential users of the information generated by it and furthermore has no control over the providers of data input to the system. This is by far the least desirable category.

The second observation I made in reviewing HISs was that the most successful were usually based primarily on *administrative* types of input data, such as those routinely collected for administrative purposes, for example, data on admission and discharge, and other items often linked to the reporting requirements determined by the funding agency. This contrasts with the many difficulties encountered in designing medically oriented national HISs with data inputs based on patients' assessments or diagnoses, for which it is very difficult to have the professionals (physicians and others) who provide these types of data agree on a uniform set of definitions and level of detail. (This is especially true of the assessment of the health status of the elderly, due to its multidimensional nature.) Another problem with this type of data is that the information the data providers are supposed to report (i.e. diagnoses) is often unknown, or only known with uncertainty at the time it is supposed to be reported on, e.g. diagnosis on admission to hospital.

What, then, are the main implications of the HIS literature review for the design of a national information system for long-term care? My personal recommendations are:

1. Ensure that potential users of the system have direct control over the HIS and are involved in its design. This is not an easy task in practice because of the

multiplicity of ministries and voluntary organizations involved in long-term care.

2. Start with an HIS based on routinely collected (or administrative-type) data. In other words, when building up your HIS try, at first, to change data reporting requirements by the long-term care service system as little as possible. Only after the data providers get used to the computerized HIS will you be able to enlarge its scope in a modular manner.

And finally an obvious comment, but maybe the most important one: the HIS in return will have to give something to the data providers to ensure their cooperation. This could be new information generated by the HIS, but not available before, and useful to the data provider; or training or explanation sessions in a pleasant environment; or even feedback on mistakes in the data given by the data providers. Any method that takes the data provider into consideration and convinces him or her that the data he gives will be used will result in smoother functioning of the new HIS.

3. OECD Experiences with the Initiation and Coordination of Health Indicator Systems, with Special Emphasis on Interinstitutional Coordination and Comparability

Jean-Pierre Poullier*

The OECD data watch of health indicators, though still in an early stage of development, is grounded on an explicit theory of the political functions of social reporting. An all-embracing health accounting approach has guided the entire effort. It has proceeded, unlike most institutional data collation exercises, through a "massaging" of national routine data processed at the centre rather than through questionnaires, but with a strong interaction between the national data agencies and the estimator (resulting in the availability of much hitherto unaccessible information). As for comparability, considerable stress has been laid on reconstructing aggregates from detailed sub-aggregates; more emphasis has been put on trends than on levels because precision is not yet attainable; large differences reflect probably real world variations, not statistical inconsistencies. Numbers can – independently of the analysis which they will ultimately serve – tell a story. Some trends not observed till today have probably a considerable relevance for policy interpretation; a few are shown, centred on price disparities and dispersions in the quantities consumed or inputs utilized. The lack of output indicators – still considered premature at the international and even national level – is a major gap in the data system, but some progress has been achieved.

The Reporting Nature of OECD's Data Watch

Though fairly modest in size and very recent, the work of OECD in the health area may be viewed as grounded on explicit theories of the political functions of social reporting. Social scientists sometimes confine this reporting role to a *factual contribution* to the political debate about the well-being of citizens, a description of "how things are" (this approach underpins *The OECD List of Social Indicators*, 1982, and a companion volume of data putting the model to the test[1]). "How things ought to be" is conventionally viewed as a judgement worked out by the political process, which, however, many analysts ignore in their technical role.

"What ought to be done" about the contrast between how things are and how they ought to be is essentially a judgement worked out by the political process, though one involving a considerable amount of technical assistance: the evaluative per-

---

* Jean-Pierre Poullier is associated with the Organisation for Economic Co-operation and Development, Paris. The opinions expressed in this contribution do not necessarily reflect those of the OECD.

1 OECD: *Living Conditions in OECD Countries*, Paris 1986

spective of policy-making implies knowledge about the conditions in which change may be implemented, about the interaction of multiple agents intervening in the process, and about the identification of the financial intermediation involved. Data – quantitative and other – about "why certain outcomes are different over time or between regions" should thus also be viewed as a *factual contribution* to the political debate about well-being when they are essentially observations or descriptions.

In an international setting, the regional dimension of social reporting becomes "nations" and the time profile can be two or more reference years or single-year observations relating to a group of countries in different stages of maturity as measured by income per head and selected institutional and resource endowment parameters. Delivery processes and output of services are particularly difficult to quantify when they are not largely provided by market mechanisms and not facing the test of productivity; health particularly has been labelled as "comparison resistant"[2] and absolute measures of efficiency or effectiveness are few and partial. When, however, a wide range of intercountry variations in the prices paid for specific services, in the quantities supplied, in the resources consumed for similar throughput, in the attainment of significant social outcomes, etc., points to large differences between one delivery system and others, the width of this difference can be turned into a "proxy" indicator to provide relative measures of efficiency or effectiveness which can be of considerable relevance to domestic policy analysts. A critical evaluation of such a new instrument still in the process of development is premature; what follows is thus more a brief presentation of parameters which have guided this process and a discussion of solutions adopted to overcome certain hurdles rather than a theoretical evaluation of the merits and limitations of alternative comparative techniques. The emphasis of the OECD data work in health has been more to demonstrate empirically that implicit mini-health accounts already exist, rather than to add to an array of accounting models – perhaps conceptually superior, but with few data in the cells of the model tables. Nevertheless, a conceptual framework has guided the estimator. We have relied heavily on A. Foulon's "Proposals for a homogeneous treatment of health expenditure in the national accounts" (*The Review of Income and Wealth*, March 1982, pp 45-70) – except that these proposals entail the production of new information in most countries and the pragmatic nature of the OECD exercise required us to work with what was already available. Also, as indicated below, the verification of plausibility and the estimation of missing values has partly been done from non-monetary data which are not part of the framework proposed by Foulon.

In Search of an Adequate Health Accounting Framework

Crudely stated, the concern of policy-makers in developing countries consists in maximizing medical outcomes with very limited inputs; in industrialized countries it has become one of optimizing considerable resources consumed in the health care process. Sophisticated health accounting systems are thus daughters of necessity

---

2 See, in particular, I.B. Kravis: *Comparative Studies of National Incomes and Prices*, and R. Marris: Comparing the incomes of nations. *The Journal of Economic Literature*, March 1984

and are mainly a development of the late 1970s.[3] The principal sets of information on which health policies rest comprise:

1. Clinical and biological data
2. Epidemiological data
3. Health status, behavioural and environmental data
4. Activity and throughput data, including resources
5. Financial (expenditure and revenue) data
6. Social protection data

Each set is composed of a number of subsets comprising a variable number of indicators, depending on perceived country needs and existing recording systems.

Most countries' health accounts are typically money flow accounts. Activity and throughput data or social protection data notably need not be part of the broader concept, because the expenditure sub-components are deemed to rest on unique or quasi-identical definitions of medical manpower and facilities, of modes of remuneration, of the earnings basis of employers' and employees' contributions, etc. When crossing national boundaries, these parameters and many others have sometimes as many interpretations and estimating methodologies as there are countries involved; reasonable consistency and comprehensiveness cannot be achieved without a minimum amount of cross-checking using non-monetary estimates. These also include a few medical data sub-sets, because some observed differences in the level of or trends in health expenditure appear directly related to natural differences in the epidemiological status of populations or in societal choices about available therapies.

Thus, for technical reasons, the comparative accounting system in progress at OECD embraces these different sets. Priorities have dictated the concentration of efforts on the socio-economic rather than the medical dimensions of health policy; virtually no clinical or biological and few epidemiological data have been collated (as the most immediate needs do not include, for instance, cost-benefit analyses of selected therapies or priority criteria for funding pharmaceutical research and, where used, shifts in morbidity patterns or the concentration of medical outlays were only taken as facts). The development of a virtual satellite account to the macro- economic accounts with a fair amount of non-monetary data and a certain neglect of medical data finds justification as a short-term opportunity cost more than in theoretical considerations. While the macro-economic facets of health policy have historically received more attention than the micro-economic side, the health economics profession is currently placing increasing emphasis on technical tools requiring more disaggregated data. This is already somewhat reflected in the present OECD health data bank designed to help analysts in their efforts to identify fundamental differences in the health delivery systems. The main emphasis of the work, however, has been to understand the "how" and "why" of large intercountry differences in spending patterns.

---

3 See Levy, E. (ed): La Santé Fait des Comptes: Une Perspective Internationale/Accounting for Health: An International Survey. *Economica*, Paris 1982

The uniqueness of the OECD exercise lies perhaps less in the conceptual all-encompassing structure of the mini-health accounts established – this can be found in a more "deconcentrated" way in several national statistical systems – than in an attempt to bypass, at the international level, conceptual procrastination through a demonstration exercise based on international conventions of classification such as the Systems of National Account (SNA) and the International Classification of Diseases (ICD). Some 80 basic tables, spanning the period 1960-1983 and covering the 24 OECD countries as far as possible, and lending themselves to perhaps as many derived comparative tables, have already been compiled. Although theoretically only a coordination of previously existing statistics, this effort may be credited with a stimulative impact on national administrations monitoring health services. The issues of coordination and comparability need perhaps to be addressed now, starting with available alternatives.

Alternative Processes of International Data Collation

A number of avenues are open when international comparisons are required. Surveys can be designed at the centre through an elaborate process, sometimes including the financing of the data collection process to assure an even higher degree of homogeneity and harmony; a small number of surveys conducted by the Statistical Office of the European Community belongs to this class. Other international agencies have lacked the political will and/or the financial resources to do likewise.

A more widely used approach consists in the adoption of a common questionnaire, based on agreed concepts, definitions and nomenclatures. These are regularly refined and are more numerous with each edition of these "comparative" yearbooks as, with the passage of time, countries integrate in their domestic reporting mechanisms a larger number of "common" guidelines. The "questionnaire approach" can be credited with considerable achievements. Integrity in the setting of a scientific colloquium demands, however, that these achievements be qualified with important reservations. It is the case that reporting systems primarily serve "domestic" administrative needs, with international questionnaires constituting a supplementary tier often filled in by careful adjustment of the "national" records which do not fully match the requirements of the "international" reporting system. International agencies have not always facilitated the task of national administrations by issuing questionnaires on identical topics with heterogeneous definitions. OECD questionnaires generally adopt the norms of the United Nations statistical system or, when none are available for the problem at hand, and always in the case of health indicators, use European Community statistical standards. Filling out international questionnaires implies a considerable commitment of national administrations; this resource is often not available in the early stages of comparative work, if only because the expected benefits of allocating scarce statistical manpower to this task appear modest until actual analyses give prominence to this effort. Even the best-known international harmonization exercises, such as national accounting and labour force statistics, comprise a fair amount of approximation – due to shortages of staff and survey money to iron out all known hurdles –

after three decades of efforts by many, both in the national agencies and the institutions coordinating these efforts.

In international organizations, as in academic research centres, the fastest way to elaborate "reasonably" comparative statistical systems remains the massaging of national data sets in order to obtain the best set of "homogeneous" time series attainable with the resources deployed, within a stated time frame, from published material. Academic researchers interact mainly with foreign colleagues to verify their work; international civil servants benefit from the cooperation of national civil servants committed to the same objective, who at times allow access to hitherto unpublished material of value to this process. While the process rests on a fair amount of approximation ex post, it involves also a rigorous effort to adapt existing data (previously published or not) to "common" technical requirements. Though this second-tier data generation is practised as a cunning method, its value should not be underestimated. Speed is an unquestionable asset: concern over runaway health expenditure would probably have become an historical event before a genuine international reporting system could be implemented. Moreover, the massaging approach may exert a strong "persuasion" effect on national agencies, particularly in smaller countries which cannot as easily as larger ones devote considerable resources to statistical standards. As the initial estimator is heavily influenced by the most elaborate reporting systems at hand, his or her work serves to reveal indicators used in those countries and, in countries with less sophisticated data systems, stimulates the supply of data and information not previously readily accessible. Even in more advanced countries, the need for statistical information commonly used elsewhere (but virtually ignored in those countries) may become acute when making an international comparison; that information then joins the list of minimum domestic data requirements.

Few countries possess comprehensive, consistent and systematic health accounts. During the on-going comparative OECD health exercise, two additional countries have taken formal steps towards the establishment of health accounting systems and another one has developed an integrated accounting approach to supplement its previous piecemeal presentation. Other countries are enlarging their domestic "health facts" publication. The requirements for detailed intercountry comparisons, to closely link monetary and non-monetary indicators, are in some respects so novel in a purely national setting that none of the 24 OECD countries assembles in a *single* yearbook or similar publication all the numerical information deemed relevant to ensure comparability, consistency and easy interpretability of observed differences; indirectly, the conduct of the OECD exercise has stimulated the release, and in some cases, the production of new data. Notwithstanding its merits and achievements, the massaging approach is one fraught with conceptual and definitional problems; these are unlikely to be eliminated in the present decade. Thus, great attention must be paid by users to the warning notes, and more concern should probably be given to time trends than to comparisons in levels, in spite of considerable breaks in national time series.

The Comparability Criterion

Health accounting in the 1980s resembles the macro-economic national accounting process of the early 1950s, including the need for the secretariat of the Organisation for European Economic Cooperation (OEEC) – the institution preceding the OECD – to develop preliminary national accounts for some countries on the basis of partial evidence. Biases in the estimating methodologies of the series partly developed by the secretariat are inherently highly consistent between countries. Centrally estimated series are regularly diminishing in number, however, just as national accounts have rapidly been fully supplied by national estimators. On the whole, official data that were previously inaccessible and which replace preliminary estimates calculated centrally on the basis of partial information are of the same order of magnitude. The estimating criteria have been different in the various sections of the present data base and cannot all be repeated here (sources and methods fill over 80 pages). The use of agreed sub-strata for each data set – agreements gradually reached over the past 30 years – ensures a fair amount of comparability. These include the joint United Nations OECD guidelines for national income accounting, the World Health Organization International Classification of Diseases and the Nordic Council on Medicines (in particular, its pioneering work to establish common reporting standards for pharmaceuticals). We are well aware of the pitfalls of comparisons at a disaggregate level (for example, mortality data from a few countries do not list bronchitis as a cause of death because the medical schools in those countries do not teach that this ailment sometimes has a fatal outcome and, consequently, other respiratory diseases include also death due to bronchitis). Micro-incomparabilities are found in all data systems, but they affect only little, if at all, the broad trends of the mini-health accounts being built up. The procedure selected has precluded a questioning of agreed-upon conventions; the only exception is the SNA rule allocating military, prison or school health services to Defence, Justice or Education, a rule not generally adhered to, which is challenged on conceptual grounds. Apparent inconsistencies in data sets are signalled to national authorities and result occasionally in the supply of substitute data deemed to better correspond to the underlying concepts of the series retained. The comparative process helps to reveal some lacunae in existing national practices and highlights procedures familiar to one or two countries, but not adopted in most.

Adherence to established conventions is particularly important for comparison of the main aggregates, since these are subject to more popular attention (e.g. tables purporting to measure the share of health expenditure to GDP or life expectancy at birth). Since no international health accounting system has been adopted to date, the OECD approach has been to select the medical care components of national accounts' reporting to establish levels of total and public expenditure on health. (A drawback of this empirical approach, for example, includes the allocation of medical services in the army to Defence rather than to Health, or the treatment of in-situ medical centres on the employer's premises as intermediate. The exclusions do not create major distortions in the absolute level of medical care spending – on average 3 percentage points where it has been possible to estimate them and of one-tenth of 1% in the ratio of health spending to GDP.) The largest disadvantage results from the fact that national accounts do not systematically disaggregate medical care into institutional care, ambulatory care, pharmaceutical consumption, etc.; this breakdown has thus to be borrowed from other data sets established along other criteria and boundaries.

Considerable progress in comparability should be attained when national accountants systematically disaggregate medical care into subfunctions and produce consolidated sets; the required will to do so is still internationally flickering and fails in the statistical world to reflect the deep concern for health expenditure growth prevailing in the "political process". Illustrations of lacunae and departures from agreed concepts are too numerous to be here listed exhaustively and are widely documented in the OECD health data watch[4].

Much the same procedure applies when measuring physical indicators. Average length of stay in hospitals conceals a large number of off-setting errors. When measured at a finer level of breakdown (such as by diagnosis) fourfold or fivefold between-countries differences for similar diseases cannot be discarded easily as variations in recording procedures. The OECD test of comparability has relied more on highlighting the plausibility or implausibility of "macro-aggregates" by use of a wide array of sub-aggregates, including the marriage of relevant monetary and non-monetary indicators, than on assembling data scrupulously respecting ICD or other relevant statistical guidelines.

Most basic series retained, or partly estimated, rest on a principle of minimum respect of statistical conventions. As may be suspected, these are often ignored for financial or institutional reasons. For instance, readmissions to hospital for the same cause occurring within a fortnight of a discharge should be linked to the previous episode and thus the original admission and the readmission counted as one; for administrative convenience, or to avoid a hidden penalty associated with very long length of stay, this convention is frequently ignored. Changing medical technology, such as a dissociation of the diagnostic from the surgical or therapeutic phases of treatment, and often also convalescence and follow-up treatment, is another cause of multiple admissions recorded for a single episode. The referral of a patient to several hospitals for different phases of a therapeutic course counts as several admissions, but the referral to several departments of a large hospital counts as one admission (it may be noted that this convention is usually not applied to outpatient services, each one being a separate contact).

From evidence readily accessible, it does not appear that published data are systematically and critically evaluated in each country. International reporting cannot remove lack of implementation of already agreed upon conventions, but, in pointing to the consequences of hazy guidelines in comparing actual country experiences, international reporting encourages a stricter implementation of statistical conventions or the adoption of more practical alternatives. The departures from conventions, however, should not be exaggerated either; one cannot discard all intercountry tables as being "non-comparable". Micro-surveys conducted by investigators able to apply equivalent standards confirm the existence of very large differences in country practices which macro-comparisons have identified.

---

[4] OECD: *Measuring Health Care 1960-1983*, Paris 1985

The "learning-by-doing" process underlining the on-going OECD exercise serves, according to some of its critics, an important coordinating function: international comparisons highlighting sizeable differences in the observation of similar medical processes are interpreted by experts as statistically implausible (leading to a questioning of the underlying conventions) or as indicators of plausible real world differences. The "political processes" involved often smoothly reduce or iron out these real differences; this is illustrated by an example in pricing relativities first identified in OECD's 1977 *Public Expenditure on Health*, now considerably diminished (Table 1).

Less visibly than real world differences may be erased, statistical conventions become somewhat more homogeneously applied through empirical exercises because many deviations from the norm were unintended; statisticians as well as analysts appreciate that no superstructure of progress can be built without an infrastructure of truth. The learning-by-doing approach is thus not antagonistic to conceptual exercises undertaken under the joint leadership of the United Nations Conference of European Statisticians and the World Health Organization, and at the Statistical Office of the European Communities. Notwithstanding this important cross-fertilization, still and probably for many years to come, there remains a considerable amount of incomparability across countries. This situation matters, it seems, more at the micro-levels of observation than at the macro-levels: offsetting trends conceal part of the underlying aggregate differences. In any case, macro differences may be so large that, even if partly accounted for by non-comparable statistical elements, they provide a relevant policy indicator of concern. The social reporting function of "How things are" leaves then the foreground to the political process of "How things ought to be". The reporting function should, however, whether repeated as a central "massaging" approach or upgraded to a more routine "questionnaire" approach, vastly improve in quality and reliability in successive endeavours.

Can Numbers Tell a Story?

The Keynesian wisdom "economists are prisoners of some defunct philosopher" applies to the search for internationally comparable statistical evidence to support international comparative economics. This process is not haphazard. Series are not selected to support a particular thesis, but they are the quantitative facet of the fundamental characteristics of economics as a science. If economics is the art of allocating scarce resources, comparative tables may be expected to exhibit the behaviour of the prices of medical services or the quantities consumed or the efficiency with which inputs are combined for stated outputs. Political concern in health policy stems mainly from rapidly rising expenditure trends and from intercountry differences in the shares of national expenditure devoted to medical care.

The starting point of the health data bank has thus been an attempt to determine more precisely the amounts spent on medical care in each country. Some conceptual problems in this respect have already been alluded to and, as indicated above, are described in a fair amount of detail in the underlying sources and methods.

Table 1. Index of selected medical services in six countries 1981[a]

Medical or paramedical services	Belgium	Denmark	France	Germany	Luxembourg	Switzerland	Average index (6 countries)	SD
Microscopic urine exam	0.38	0.37	0.14[b]	0.83	0.21	0.51	0.40	0.25
Extraction grinder	1.22	1.72	1.50	1.78	0.61	0.65	1.25	0.52
Home attendance by general practioner	1.37	1.48	1.2	3.48	1.42	1.51	1.74	0.86
X-ray unit (2 negatives)	1.90	2.24	1.17	3.1	0.58	2.12	1.89	0.91
Electrophorese	1.53	0.74	1.96	2.97	1.07	1.71	1.66	0.78
Electroencephalogram	7.31	3.69	9.20	9.58	2.26	10.54	7.10	3.39
Bilateral amygdalectomy on a child under 10 years	5.87	–	5.52	10.3	7.25	12.04	8.20	2.86
Normal confinement pre- and post-natal care	15.25	7.75	14.36	7.66	–	12.26	11.46	3.59
Scintigraphy of thyroid	11.14	–	–	7.80	3.80	1.54	6.07	4.26
Total tooth prosthesis (one jaw)	22.0	–	15.98	40.09	28.8	–	26.72	10.34
Trepanation brain abcess by neurosurgeon	25.5	–	14.72	25.08	41.87	23.29	26.09	9.84
Anaesthesia by specialist for stereotaxia	63.77	–	20.24	(5.63)	26.18	–	36.73	23.60
Intracardial surgery under hypothermy	90.33	–	46.0	104.52	–	199.14	110.0	64.44
Memorandum: Fee for general practicioner at beginning of 1981 (in national currency)	FB 244	DK 48.81	FF 50	DM 8.15	FL 429	Max SF 23.25 Min SF 8.20	–	–

Sources: Calculated from International Association for Mutual Assistance, Document issu de la Commission pour l'Etude du Problème des Relations avec le Corps Medical, Geneva, 1981, mimeo

[a] Consultation of general practitioner = 1 in each country

[b] Min

Expenditures have been disaggregated first into their public and private components, next into the main health subfunctions (institutional care, ambulatory care, pharmaceuticals, therapeutic appliances – with all sets measured for total and public expenditure). The interest of this disaggregation has a conceptual as well as a statistical dimension. The latter lies, obviously, in a better apprehension of the components of medical spending and gives rise to considerable adjustments in spending totals. (In a very recent international comparison of health expenditure trends there were nearly as many expenditure concepts as countries retained. For instance, the classic German health accounts include "Barleistungen" (payments in cash), whereas cash transactions are elsewhere normally classified under social insurance; the same thing happens for rehabilitation outlays, which are sometimes classified under medical care, but often as welfare outlays.) Conceptually, disaggregation allows better comparisons of service intensity measured in expenditure flows; intensity is larger where hospital care is more prevalent than ambulatory care. Without much analysis, data sets explain away a sizeable part of the differences noted in the usual tables as structural differences or as statistical variations which the political process comments and to which it reacts. The implicit OECD tables which exclude already a sizeable amount of statistical incomparabilities are expected to ease the analyst's work, leaving him to explain the most substantive intercountry variations. All analyses concur in attributing to general inflation a substantial role in the expansion of medical expenditure. The data assembled permit to measure the impact of the medically specific role of inflation for each subfunction. These trends are particularly important since – notwithstanding the rising importance of hospitals which experience in most years above average price increases – medically specific inflation rates have decelerated in the 1970s compared with the 1960s and this decelerating trend appears to extend into the 1980s (Table 2).

National data systems need not necessarily integrate several data sets to assist the analytical process in providing information (say, on the number of services performed on average per physician to substantiate in part a first hypothesis, and institutional data on income freeze and income restraint measures adopted to substantiate a second). A comparative data system which does not supply such evidence rapidly becomes barren. The OECD data bank is still very primitive, but series available suggest that neither of the two hypotheses referred to above appears incongruous, or unique to a particular country. Admittedly, a statistical display is not sufficient proof and further analysis is required. A "data watch" may be designed to pursue the objective of providing very detailed information to answer the question of "Why things are" before helping the political process question of "What ought to be done".

The political process may require rather simple abstractions though some difficult ethical ones; the technical process is a complex one, to which an organized data system contributes increased stability. A continuous flow of reasonably consistent trends relating to a large number of countries may help to interpret individual country trends. Some examples indicate that the build-up of international series has stimulated the release of additional evidence hitherto little used in a national setting only and to relativize member countries' observed positions.

Table 2. Absolute and relative price trends in institutional care (average annual growth in percentage points)

	Absolute hospital price rises			Hospital specific price rises		
	1960-70	1970-80	1977-82[a]	1960-70	1970-80	1977-82[a]
Australia	–	–	–	–	–	–
Austria	12.87	12.38	10.80	3.42	1.96	1.54
Belgium	9.39	8.99	7.49	2.74	1.26	1.49
Canada	6.42	11.01	11.13	2.15	1.23	1.13
Denmark	15.22	10.72	12.21	2.39	1.12	1.31
Finland	6.91	11.64	10.24	1.20	1.01	1.12
France	6.34	10.56	10.71	1.44	1.11	0.95
Germany	9.11	8.67	7.30	2.51	1.66	1.69
Greece	5.50	23.76	27.31	1.74	1.72	1.47
Ireland	14.35	14.01	10.07	2.67	1.01	0.72
Italy	16.43	16.53	18.79	3.62	1.11	1.08
Japan	8.25	12.25	3.56	1.54	1.51	0.79
Netherlands	13.53	8.14	8.52	2.56	1.06	1.60
New Zealand	5.87	15.58	10.24	1.50	1.18	0.69
Norway	8.19	8.95	9.44	1.68	1.06	0.92
Portugal	–	18.35	25.54	–	1.15	1.27
Sweden	8.40	12.49	5.95	2.00	1.29	0.63
Switzerland	–	1.80	7.40	–	0.34	1.64
United Kingdom	5.51	18.03	14.68	1.31	1.28	1.14
United States	4.88	8.62	10.53	1.63	1.23	1.28

Medically specific inflation trends can be supplemented by evidence about earnings in the medical professions, showing a decline in relativities for physicians and dentists. These developments and their underlying causes need be interpreted, notably the relative importance of (a) competitive pressures generated by increasing number of professionals (and some slowdown in consumption growth), and (b) public policy to regulate professional incomes (or professional self-restraint to prevent regulatory action on incomes).

[a] last 5 years if 1977-82 not available

Regarding the volume of medical services consumed, the OECD health data watch has purposely moved away from classic stock indicators, used in most international comparisons (such as hospital beds or physicians per 1000 inhabitants), in favour of throughput indicators: bed-days per person per year, number of medicines consumed per person per year, etc. Stock indicators fail to depict real consumption of services or, at least, their true intensity in the delivery process; they are, however, useful to interpret throughput measures. There is, for example, a mechanical relationship between an endowment of hospital beds and the average length of stay in hospitals. The priorities given to the build-up of statistical tables, by and large, have been dictated both by wide availability of the basic series and a probability that they would provide quantitative explanations of intercountry differentials.

Throughput indicators improve on stock measures, but remain imperfect measures of volume. First, they may conceal opposite real world developments, such as increasing admission rates and declining length of stay (in a comparison of levels, countries displaying low admission rates and high length of stay may have a similar value for bed-days per person as countries displaying high admission rates and low length of stay). In addition, these sub-aggregates are subject to differences in demographic structures of countries (the elderly typically record longer inpatient spells) and in their prevailing morbidity patterns. The process of disaggregation by age, sex and disease categories is far from complete, but the tables achieved distill percussive information about real differences in average country practices: length of stay may be a poor absolute indicator, but it is a powerful relative measurement. It will be interesting to review the intercountry differences in the latter part of the 1980s (Table 3).

The search for performance indicators in health systems has been at the forefront of policy concern in the past decades due to growing financial constraints. Widely accepted indicators are few in OECD countries and thus even fewer in a comparative framework, though some measures with only limited absolute significance may yield relevant questions in a relative setting. A considerable part of the observed intercountry differences in the level of resources allocated to the health industry is accounted for by differences in the relative pricing of medical services and in the relative demand for these services, as much as in quantities of inputs involved in their supply. Evidence at hand indicates that intercountry disparities remain considerable in spite of the convergence observed for some indicators. Data (not supplied here because the present status of tabulation attained is too fragmentary to suggest a similar generalization) point, however, to much higher surgical rates and/or relative unit costs in the countries with the highest relative spending ratios. The process of data collection of characteristics pertinent to the description of "comparison resistant services", helps to reduce the resistance to comparisons but it also stimulates cross-fertilization in the search for output measures in single countries.

Health Status Indicators as Proxies for Output Measures

The quest for a comprehensive index of population health status much predates the general concern for health expenditure which, in turn, has generated consistent and systematic health accounts in a number of countries. Over the years, many general indexes have been proposed. OECD has greatly advanced a conceptual consensus that "ways of linking both life expectancy and expected disability of healthy persons to causes of death and disability are a crucial step in establishing the usefulness of social indicators for policy planning and evaluation".[5] Experts have, however, shied away from translating this concept into an operational OECD Social Indicator. Life expectancy thus continues to be a standard gauge, glossing over the 15% of life spent by individuals on average in long-term institutions or in serious states of disability.

---

5 OECD: *Measuring Social Well-Being*, pp. 62-63, Paris 1976

Table 3. Varations in somatic hospital mean length-of-stay by disease categories, 1980[a]

ICD class	Disease category	Average[b] (days)	Lowest (days)	Range		
				Ratio (days)	Highest to lowest index	Standard deviation[b]
1.	Infectious and parasitic diseases	14.0	5.8	20.3	4.5	5.5
2.	Neoplasms	15.0	10.5	15.2	4.1	2.6
3.	Endocrine and metabolic diseases	15.8	9.6	10.8	2.1	3.9
4.	Diseases of the blood	11.9	5.0	30.9	7.1	6.6
6.	Diseases of the nervous system	16.8	5.4	31.4	6.8	8.7
7.	Diseases of the circulatory system	19.4	9.7	21.4	3.2	6.5
8.	Diseases of the respiratory system	10.1	4.8	12.3	3.6	3.3
9.	Diseases of the digestive system	10.6	6.7	8.4	2.3	2.9
10.	Diseases of the genito-urinary system	8.9	5.1	18.5	4.6	4.0
11.	Complications of pregnancy and childbirth	6.0	2.5	6.6	3.6	2.1
12.	Diseases of the skin and subcutaneous tissue	11.5	6.9	11.1	2.6	3.7
13.	Diseases of the musculo-skeletal system and connective tissue	15.3	8.3	11.5	2.85	4.1
14.	Congenital anomalies	11.4	6.6	9.4	2.4	2.7
15.	Certain causes of perinatal morbidity and mortality	11.6	4.6	14.4	4.1	4.3
16.	Symptoms or ill-defined conditions	10.2	4.5	16.6	4.7	-
17.	Accidents, poisoning and violence	11.6	7.7	12.0	2.6	3.8

[a] 19 countries average, excluding Belgium, Iceland, Luxembourg, Portugal and also Japan (which has not been included in the calculation, as its in-patient care practice varies in many ways from that of the most other countries).

[b] In a few countries the data relate to a year before 1980; this leads to a small overestimate of the range.

Source: OECD: *Measuring Health Care 1960-1983*, Paris 1985, p. 16

While the more classic measures are still prevalent, the OECD data watch has attempted to depart from conventional wisdom in placing more emphasis on morbidity than on mortality data. This choice is dictated by huge advances in life-saving medical technologies, leaving larger shares of the population wholly or partially disabled. Failing (at this stage) to provide a comprehensive health status index, the OECD data watch has focused on partial indicators of victimization and morbidity, etc. with an expected outcome: man-made morbidity is fast overtaking natural morbidity as the main cause of the increasing use of the medical system.

The information is, however, not geared wholly on the biological outcome, but on the social processes themselves, since, for instance, it may have been little observed that, in virtually all countries, the prices of consumption goods with well-known adverse effects on human health have increased less rapidly than those of all consumer goods and services. For most analysts, the paucity of readily available information explains perhaps a relative neglect of behavioural and environmental factors in the growth of health expenditures.

A Provisional State

Beyond a putative factual contribution to document rising outlays, however, there would be no neutral social reporting process if it did not highlight also profound changes brought about by the success of medical care in dramatically reducing premature mortality and indirect productivity losses through shorter disease spells. Longitudinal cost-of-illness accounting is only experimental, but the results suggest that the invisible gains of the visible costs of disease may well outweigh the high cost of the system. OECD cannot at the centre generate cost-of-illness accounts for its countries, but in diffusing the experience of smaller countries whose languages are less accessible it has helped stimulate the growth of evidence about the benefits of health systems.

As a conclusion to these introductory remarks on hidden principles and guidelines of international health care comparisons, consider the idea that without a formal systems science theory behind it, the OECD comparative data system has respected many features of systems analysis: an attempt at comprehensiveness, an attempt at consistency, an attempt at integrating several dimensions of the problem even if economics has been privileged. Admittedly, this is only a beginning and the road is still long before full-fledged all-embracing comparisons will become possible; gaps remain important and surrogates too many. The initial objective, given the specificity of OECD in socio-economic policy analysis, has been one of identifying the main money flows accruing to medical care, as national authorities have; however, the task has rapidly proven impossible without integrating a considerable number of non-monetary variables in this national satellite account framework. Genuine international comparisons in health expenditure may still be a decade away; however, the task looks somewhat less formidable than it did two or three years ago, thanks notably to experts in statistical agencies who critically reviewed the initial effort. This achievement should not be overstated: if it is only a one-of-a-kind exercise, the "persuasion" and "massaging" benefits will largely vanish. Only repeated harmonization exercises will assure a lasting and deepening effect.

4. Health Surveillance in Europe: An Indicator-Based Reporting System

Karen Davis*

In September 1984 the European Region of the World Health Organization adopted a set of health targets to be achieved by member states by the year 2000. This sets the stage for a major focus on strategies for achieving improved health outcomes in industrialized nations. One step in accomplishing this effort is the development of an indicator-based monitoring system. This system should make it possible to pinpoint major health problems, analyze health indicator variations across countries and over time with a view to identifying the determinants of better performance, and monitor future trends.

An indicator-based reporting system could be used as a broad-scale health surveillance system. A parallel can be found in the case regarding contagious diseases, where a reporting system of contagious disease outbreaks or "hot spots" can concentrate efforts of public health officers. Similarly, a reporting system that includes indicators on chronic conditions, accidents, infant and maternal mortality, health risks related to lifestyles, the work place, and the environment, and other health problems common to industrialized nations can serve as a health surveillance system to draw attention to "hot spots" that require the concentrated efforts of public health officials to combat.

This paper (a) briefly describes the development of the European Regional health targets; (b) reports on a microcomputer software package developed by the author for WHO-EURO to demonstrate health indicator data relating to these targets; (c) describes the preliminary health indicator data base currently available including statistics from a wide variety of official WHO studies and documents, as well as studies and reports published by other organizations and individuals; (d) presents some information on variations in health indicators across European countries, historical trends, and future projections based on historical trends using the microcomputer software package; and (e) discusses the potential utility of such an indicator-based system.

---

* Karen Davis, Ph.D., is Chairman and Professor, Department of Health Policy and Management, School of Hygiene and Public Health, Johns Hopkins University, Baltimore. The views expressed are those of the author and not necessarily those of the World Health Organization or Johns Hopkins University.

World Health Organization: European Regional Targets

In May 1977 the World Health Organization World Health Assembly adopted a resolution that "the main social target of governments and WHO in the coming decades should be the attainment by all citizens of the world by the year 2000 of a level of health that will permit them to lead a socially and economically productive life" [6]. Commonly called the "Health For All by the Year 2000" resolution, this resolution has been the guiding framework for the development of WHO strategies and programs. Each region of the World Health Organization was urged to develop specific strategies for achieving this goal.

At the regional committee meeting of the European Region of WHO in 1980, member states approved their first common health policy – a European strategy for attaining health for all by the year 2000 [7]. The need for this strategy was based on a recognition of two basic facts:

1. Despite substantial health expenditures and application of sophisticated technology, the health status of the population was clearly below achievable levels.
2. Despite the high level of economic, educational, and scientific development in the region, unacceptable inequalities in health outcomes and resources persisted.

Given the advanced state of economic and scientific development common to the European member states, the European Health For All Strategy embraced four main areas of concern: lifestyles and health, risk factors affecting health and the environment, reorientation of the health care system, and mechanisms for achieving health improvements, including political, management, technological, manpower, research, and other support.

To give teeth to this common health policy, the member states further committed themselves to bringing country health policies and programming into line with the health for all strategy and to report on progress toward achieving this strategy every 2 years beginning in 1983, and a thorough evaluation every 6 years beginning in 1985.

This unprecedented agreement inaugurated a new era not only of increased commitment to achieving improved health of the population, but also a spirit of international solidarity to share national experiences, information, and progress among countries through a common reporting framework.

In September 1984, the member states of the European Region took a further step and formally approved a European Regional Targets document setting forth 38 specific targets to be achieved by member states by the year 2000 [8]. These targets were selected through extensive scientific working group consultation and preliminary review of the targets document at the 1983 regional committee meeting of member states. The targets may be grouped as follows:

1. *Equity in health:* Target 1 calls for reducing differences in health status between countries and within countries by at least 25% by the year 2000, by

improving the level of health of disadvantaged nations and groups.

2. *Improving health and reducing disease and its consequences:* Targets 2 through 12 are directly concerned with health improvement, including targets on life expectancy, infant mortality, maternal mortality, communicable diseases, disability, heart disease, cancer, accidents, and suicide.
3. *Promoting healthy lifestyles:* Targets 13 through 17 emphasize health promotion through health education and targets to improve positive health behavior (balanced nutrition, non-smoking, physical activity, and stress management) and reduce harmful health behavior (alcohol and drug abuse, dangerous driving, and violent social behavior).
4. *Assuring a healthy environment:* Targets 18 through 25 stress a healthy environment and safe workplace. Specific targets cover such areas as environmental risks, water and air pollution, hazardous waste, safe housing, and protection against work-related health risks.
5. *Appropriate care:* Targets 26 through 31 emphasize primary care as a route toward achieving health targets. Individual targets cover the distribution of resources, the content, coordination, and quality of care.
6. *Knowledge development and other support:* Targets 32 through 38 emphasize the need for research, health policy actions, resource allocation, health information systems, human resource development, health technology assessment, and intersectoral cooperation as supporting actions to assure attainment of the health for all strategy.

The regional committee also provisionally approved 65 essential indicators and other optional indicators which would be used to monitor progress toward these 38 targets [8]. For example, target 4 calls for reducing disease and disability. Essential indicators used to monitor this target include:

1. Number of disability days per person and per year, by level of restriction
2. Percentage of population experiencing different levels of long-term disability, by age and sex
3. Incidence of tuberculosis, intestinal infectious diseases, viral hepatitis, venereal diseases, and influenza. Optional indicators include expectation of disability-free life and incidence and/or prevalence of selected major chronic conditions

By the fall of 1984, WHO-EURO had some preliminary data that bear on 17 of the 38 targets. The data base includes data on 26 of 65 essential indicators and 8 of the optional indicators. Since each indicator may have several data items (e.g. standardized death rates for different age-sex groups), over 100 different data items are currently available for most European member states. Member states are being urged to submit data under standardized definitions on all essential indicators as part of the 1985 evaluation report.

Computer Assisted Planning Microcomputer Software Package

Under contract to the WHO European Regional Office, I developed a microcomputer software package for entering data on the health indicators, displaying the data in a graphical, tabular, and map format, and projecting future trends on the basis of historical experience. The basic purpose of the package is to encourage and promote attainment of the health targets by facilitating the monitoring of country efforts. Further, it permits sharing information and experiences among member states. Specifically, the Computer Assisted Planning (CAP) software package permits a variety of applications, including:

1. Displaying current and historical target indicator data for the European member states
2. Monitoring trends in the target indicators
3. Comparing health indicators across countries
4. Comparing health indicators across groups within countries
5. Making future projections based on historical trends and comparing these projection with specific targets to be achieved by the year 2000

The CAP software currently runs on the Apple II, the IBM-PC, and the Wang microcomputers. One element of the software package is a menu-driven graphics program. The user may select any country among the European member states (see Appendix A) as a reference country from the first menu display. Then any of the 38 targets may be selected from the second menu display (see Appendix B), and any of the indicator data items may be selected from the third menu display (see Appendix C). Finally, the user may select a choice of display formats, including colored bar charts, line graphs, maps, and rank ordered tables. Each of the chart displays shows the reference country indicator value, the average indicator value for the European region as a whole, and the highest and lowest country on that indicator. Future projections based on historical trends may also be shown, and contrasted with targets for the year 2000.

Other programs in the package permit adding new indicator data items to the data base, revising, or updating existing data items. Hard copies of tables or charts can be printed; slides can also be made for presentation without the computer. Minor modification of the software package permits using the same programs to make subnational area comparisons.

Available health indicator data relating to the 38 health targets were presented to the 1984 regional committee meeting of WHO-EURO using the CAP software package. In addition, key representatives of member states attended an orientation workshop following the regional committee meeting to become familiar with the capability of CAP for updating and revising the data base, demonstrating and analyzing health indicator variations across groups, both across European nations and across population subgroups within a given country, and monitoring future trends in the health indicators (see [3] for a detailed description of the software package and preliminary health indicator data base).

Health Indicator Data Base

As part of the CAP project, WHO-EURO staff pulled together data available in the summer of 1984 on the essential and optional health indicators for European member states. Available data at that time fell into the following categories:

1. Death rates adjusted for age and sex, disaggregated by cause and age-sex category (see [2] for details of standardized mortality data)
2. Communicable disease rates
3. Lifestyle data on cigarette consumption, alcohol consumption, illegal drug consumption, psychotropic drug consumption, food consumption, and literacy rates
4. Resources, including limited health expenditure data and supply of different health professionals and hospital capacity
5. Maternal and child care, including infant immunization rates for different conditions, low birth weight infants, birth rates, fertility rates, and abortion rates

The quality and reliability of the data are variable, and represent a starting point for further improvement. Examination of the data suggest that the death rate information is reasonably accurate, followed by information on resources, lifestyle, maternal and child care, with communicable disease rates more reflective of the comprehensiveness of reporting rather than actual incidence rates for the population. As of the fall of 1984, the data base did not include data on measures of disability, and environmental and occupational health risks. Health expenditure data were limited, but this gap in the data base should be filled by mid-1985 with inclusion of comprehensive standardized health expenditure data from the OECD.

This preliminary data base was shared with member states during the fall and winter of 1984, and member states supplied revised, updated, and additional data elements as part of the evaluation of the health for all strategy in March 1985. Thus, the health indicator data base is being continuously improved and expanded as additional information from member states becomes available.

Even at this stage, however, some interesting findings are apparent. The preliminary data point to some major areas where significant health gains are possible, suggest some tentative hypotheses about the determinants of better health indicator performance, and provide a basis for projecting future trends against which to assess the effort required to meet specified targets.

Life Expectancy

Target 6 calls for increasing the life expectancy at birth in the European region to at least 75 years. In 1980, the life expectancy at birth for males in the European region was 69.6 years, and 76.3 for women, or an average of 73 years for both sexes (calculated from WHO, 1984 as reported in [3]). Women, on average, live almost 7 years longer than men. Between 1960 and 1980, life expectancy at birth for both men and women increased by four years. Given this past trend, increasing the overall life expectancy by two years should be a feasible target. Projecting on the basis of past trends, life expectancy at birth for males would be 73.5 in the year 2000, and female life expectancy at birth would be 81.2, or an average of 77 – well in excess of the target value of 75 [3].

Table 1 indicates the variation in life expectancy at birth among the member states of the European region of WHO. In 1980, among the 26 countries reporting

Table 1. Life expectancy males; Indicator 6-1-1

Country	1960	1980	Projection
EUR	65.8	69.6	73.5
ALB	63.7	0	0
AUT	65.5	69	72.6
BEL	67.7	69.5	71.3
BUL	67.8	68.5	69.2
CZE	67.6	66.9	66.2
DDR	67.3	68.9	70.5
DEN	70.4	71.2	72.0
DEU	66.8	69.9	73.1
FIN	64.9	68.5	72.2
FRA	67.2	70.5	73.9
GRE	67.5	73.2	79.3
HUN	65.2	65.5	65.8
ICE	70.8	73.6	76.5
IRE	68.1	69.3	70.5
ITA	67.2	70.7	74.3
LUX	0	69.9	0
MAT	66.8	68.8	70.8
MON	0	0	0
MOR	0	0	0
NET	71.4	72.5	73.6
NOR	71.3	72.4	73.5
POL	64.8	66.1	67.4
POR	60.7	67.3	74.6
ROM	61.5	66.6	72.1
SMR	0	0	0
SPA	67.3	71.3	75.5
SSR	64.4	0	0
SWE	71.2	72.8	74.4
SWI	69.5	72.3	75.2
TUR	0	0	0
UNK	68.1	70.4	72.9
YUG	62.2	67.8	73.9

Source: WHO, World Health Statistics Annual.

information (out of 32 member states), 73.6 years for Iceland was the highest male life expectancy at birth, contrasted with a low of 65.5 for Hungary. That is, males born in Iceland can expect to live 8 years longer on average than males born in Hungary. Nordic countries have a relatively high male life expectancy – 71.3 in Denmark, 72.4 in Norway, and 72.8 in Sweden, although Finland is low at 68.5. Other countries with a male life expectancy at birth above 70.0 include France, Greece, Italy, the Netherlands, Spain, Switzerland, and the United Kingdom. Eastern European countries have a relatively low male life expectancy at birth – 68.5 in Bulgaria, 66.9 in Czechoslovakia, 68.9 in East Germany, 65.5 in Hungary,

Table 2. Life expectancy females; Indicator 6-1-2

Country	1960	1980	Projection
EUR	71.7	76.3	81.2
ALB	66	0	0
AUT	72	76.1	80.4
BEL	73.5	76.2	78.9
BUL	71.4	73.9	76.4
CZE	73.1	74.1	75.1
DDR	72.2	74.5	76.8
DEN	73.8	77.4	81.1
DEU	72.3	76.8	81.5
FIN	71.6	77.6	84.1
FRA	73.8	78.8	84.1
GRE	70.7	77.8	85.6
HUN	69.6	72.8	76.1
ICE	76.2	80.5	85.0
IRE	71.9	74.7	77.6
ITA	72.3	77.4	82.8
LUX	0	75.3	0
MAT	70.9	72.6	74.3
MON	0	0	0
MOR	0	0	0
NET	74.8	79.5	84.4
NOR	75.6	79.4	83.3
POL	70.5	74.6	78.9
POR	66.4	74.2	82.9
ROM	65	71.9	79.5
SMR	0	0	0
SPA	71.9	77.3	83.1
SSR	71.7	0	0
SWE	74.7	79.1	83.7
SWI	74.8	79.1	83.6
TUR	0	0	0
UNK	73.8	76.5	79.4
YUG	65.3	73.2	82.0

Source: WHO, World Health Statistics Annual.

66.1 in Poland, 66.6 in Romania, and 67.8 in Yugoslavia, with the USSR not reporting in 1980.

Female life expectancy at birth also varies considerably across the European countries (see Table 2). In 1980, Iceland had the highest female life expectancy at birth of 80.5 years while Romania had the lowest female life expectancy at birth of 71.9 years, or an 8.5-year differential. Among the highest female life expectancy countries are France at 78.8, the Netherlands at 79.5, Norway at 79.4, Sweden at 79.1, and Switzerland at 79.1. The lowest female life expectancy countries include Bulgaria at 73.9, Hungary at 72.8, Malta at 72.6, and Yugoslavia at 73.2.

Obviously, life expectancy at birth reflects a number of different factors. Life expectancy can be low, for example, because many infants die, because accidents take a large proportion of the young adult population, because heart disease fells men in middle age, or because cancer shortens the life of older adults. Other health indicators used to monitor health help to fill out this overall health picture provided by data on life expectancy at birth.

Infant Health

Infant mortality has declined markedly in Europe over the period from 1960 to 1982. In all countries reporting data in both years (24 out of 32), infant mortality declined over the period. The average for Europe as a whole dropped from 37.5 deaths per 1000 live births in 1960 to 24.9 deaths per 1000 live births in 1982 (see Table 3). (The latest infant mortality data for most countries are for 1982, although data for some countries are for 1981 or 1980.) The target agreed to by member states of WHO-EURO is reduction of the average rate to below 20 deaths per 1000 live births by the year 2000. If countries continue their past rate of decline, this target should be easily achievable by that time.

In the most recent period Finland reports the lowest infant mortality at 6.5 deaths per 1000 live births. The Nordic countries are among the lowest infant mortality countries – with Denmark at 8.2 deaths per 1000 live births, Iceland at 7.1, Norway at 8.0, and Sweden at 6.8. Other countries with infant mortality rates below 10 deaths per 1000 live births include the Netherlands at 8.3, France at 9.5, and Switzerland at 7.7. At the high end of the range, Morocco reported an infant mortality of 99 deaths per 1000 live births and Turkey 83, two developing countries that have elected to be a part of the European region of WHO. Considerable effort will be required to bring infant mortality for these two countries down to 20 deaths per 1000 live births. Other countries with infant mortality rates currently exceeding the target set for the year 2000 include Albania (43), Hungary (21), Poland (20.4), Portugal (26), Romania (28), USSR (27.7), and Yugoslavia (30.6).

In a study of low birth weight infants published in the *World Health Statistics Quarterly* in 1980 with data on 18 European countries, approximately 7.5% of all births in reporting countries were infants weighing less than 2 500 g (see Table 4). Those countries with an average below 5 percent included: Belgium (4.9%), Finland (3.9%), Malta (4.2%), the Netherlands (4%), Norway (4.2%), and Sweden (3.6%). Those with averages at 8% or higher included: Hungary (11.7%), Italy (11%), Poland (8%), and the USSR (8%).

It is interesting to note that Finland has the lowest infant mortality rate, but ranks toward the bottom on male life expectancy at birth. This suggests that health problems of men in later ages is a relatively serious problem in Finland.

Accidents

Accidents are a leading cause of death in children and younger adults, and a significant health problem for many industrialized nations. Table 5 indicates

Table 3. Infant mortality; Indicator 7-1

Country	1960	1982	Projection	Target
EUR	37.5	24.9	16.6	20
ALB	0	43	0	20
AUT	37.5	12.8	4.3	20
BEL	31.1	11.1	3.9	20
BUL	30.8	18.2	10.7	20
CZE	23.5	16.1	11.0	20
DDR	0	12.3	0	20
DEN	21.5	8.2	3.1	20
DEU	33.7	10.9	3.5	20
FIN	21.0	6.5	2.0	20
FRA	23.2	9.5	3.8	20
GRE	34.3	14.7	6.3	20
HUN	47.6	21	9.2	20
ICE	15.0	7.1	3.3	20
IRE	29.2	10.5	3.7	20
ITA	43.8	13	3.8	20
LUX	0	12.1	0	20
MAT	34.8	14.9	6.3	20
MON	0	0	0	20
MOR	0	99	0	20
NET	16.5	8.3	4.1	20
NOR	18.8	8	3.3	20
POL	56.0	20.4	7.4	20
POR	77.5	26	8.7	20
ROM	75.7	28	10.3	20
SMR	0	0	0	20
SPA	35.1	10.3	3.0	20
SSR	0	27.7	0	20
SWE	16.6	6.8	2.7	20
SWI	21.1	7.7	2.8	20
TUR	0	83	0	20
UNK	22.3	12	6.4	20
YUG	71.8	30.6	13.0	20

Source: WHO Statistical Data System.
Historical data for BUL, GRE, and YUG are for 1965, rather than 1960. Latest data for ALB, MOR, and UNK are for 1980 rather than 1982. Latest data for DDR, FIN, HUN, SPA, and YUG are for 1981 rather than 1982. Latest data for SSR are prior to 1980 rather than 1982.

standardized death rates from external causes for males ages 5 to 64. The average for the European region is 80.3 deaths per 100 000 population in the 1975-1979 period, up slightly from 77.2 deaths per 100 000 in 1955-1959. Fourteen of 25 reporting countries, or slightly more than half, reported an increased non elderly male death rate from external causes over the 20 year period. The target set by WHO-EURO member states is a 25% reduction in the accident death rate by the

Table 4. Low birth weight; Indicator 16-4

Country	1980
EUR	7.5
ALB	0
AUT	5.8
BEL	4.9
BUL	0
CZE	6.1
DDR	6.3
DEN	6.4
DEU	6.7
FIN	3.9
FRA	6.5
GRE	0
HUN	11.7
ICE	0
IRE	0
ITA	11
LUX	0
MAT	4.2
MON	0
MOR	0
NET	4
NOR	4.2
POL	8
POR	0
ROM	0
SMR	0
SPA	0
SSR	8
SWE	3.6
SWI	0
TUR	0
UNK	7
YUG	7.4

Source: World Health Statistics Quarterly Report, Vol. 33, No. 3, 1980.

year 2000. This could prove a particularly difficult target to reach, given the upward historical trend.

Again, there is considerable variation within the region on this health indicator, ranging from 132.1 in Finland to 46.2 in the Netherlands – nearly a three-fold difference. Other countries with a non-elderly male death rate from external causes exceeding 100 deaths per 100 000 population are Austria (115.6), Hungary (121.5), Luxembourg (100.4), Poland (119.7), and Portugal (110.2). Other countries with a non-elderly male death rate from external causes below 60 per 100 000

Table 5. Accidents external causes; Indicator 11-1-1

Country	1957	1977	Projection
EUR	77.2	80.3	83.6
ALB	0	0	0
AUT	126.4	115.6	105.7
BEL	78.7	78.0	77.4
BUL	65.6	81.3	100.7
CZE	93.4	98.7	104.4
DDR	0	0	0
DEN	73.5	72.0	70.5
DEU	98.6	83.8	71.2
FIN	120	132.1	145.6
FRA	102.8	95.6	89.0
GRE	47.4	54.1	61.7
HUN	93.8	121.5	157.3
ICE	105.2	95.3	86.3
IRE	38.8	61.8	98.4
ITA	69.0	59.3	50.9
LUX	132.5	100.4	76.0
MAT	23.2	33.4	48.0
MON	0	0	0
MOR	0	0	0
NET	47.6	46.2	44.7
NOR	68.7	67.2	65.8
POL	78.7	119.7	182.2
POR	72.4	110.2	167.6
ROM	65.8	94.7	136.3
SMR	0	0	0
SPA	55.4	60.3	65.6
SSR	0	0	0
SWE	76.6	82.4	88.8
SWI	104.8	85.6	69.9
TUR	0	0	0
UNK	50.4	47.5	44.9
YUG	83.0	94.4	107.3

Source: WHO-Euro Statistical Data System.
Data are age adjusted rates averaged for five years from 1955-1959 and 1960-1964. Historical data for BUL, GRE, ICE, and YUG are for 1960-1964. Historical data for LUX and MAT are for 1965-1969.

population include: Greece (54.1), Italy (59.3), Malta (33.4), and the United Kingdom (47.5).

About 40% of non-elderly male accidental deaths are attributable to motor vehicle traffic deaths. In the late 1970s motor vehicle traffic accidents claimed the lives of 32 men ages 5 to 64 per 100 000 population. Romania had the highest rate at 95 deaths per 100 000; Malta, on the other hand, reported only 7 deaths per 100 000.

Clearly, many deaths from external causes are preventable. Major efforts to reduce accidental deaths in areas with high rates will be required to achieve this particular health target.

Heart Disease

Heart disease is a major killer of middle-age men. It is typically the leading cause of death among older males. Unlike the US experience, heart disease death rates have been on the upswing in the last 20 years in many European countries. As shown in Table 6, the European regional average standardized death rate from ischemic heart disease for men ages 35 to 64 is 185 deaths per 100 000 population. Death rates are a 5-year average for the period 1975 to 1979. This rate is a substantial increase from a level of 147 deaths per 100 000 in the 5-year period from 1955 to 1959. All reporting countries except Luxembourg and Switzerland reported an increase over this period.

This suggests that attainment of the target of a 20% reduction in mortality from diseases of the circulatory system by the year 2000 should be quite difficult. In fact, if previous historical annual rates of increase continue, the ischemic heart disease death rate for males ages 35 to 64 should increase from 185 per 100 000 in the late 1970s to 232 per 100 000 in the year 2000, rather than a 20% decline to 150 per 100 000. Variations across countries on this indicator are also substantial. Finland has the highest non-elderly male heart disease death rate at 455 deaths per 100 000, contrasted with a low of 95.8 in France – more than a four-fold difference. Heart disease death rates among non-elderly males do not seem to explain the low life expectancy of Eastern European countries. Among reporting countries, Bulgaria at 161.5 deaths per 100 000, Poland at 179.2, Romania at 109.6, and Yugoslavia at 124.9 are all below the European average; while Hungary at 243.4 and Czechoslovakia at 279.9 are above the European average, but below the experience of the UK at 334.1 and Ireland at 325.4 deaths per 100 000.

Cancer

The European regional target for cancer is also quite ambitious. European member states have agreed to a target reduction in mortality from cancer in people under 65 of at least 15% of the 1980 rate by the year 2000.

Health indicator data on cancer for the member states of the European region show a mixed picture. Cancer death rates for men under age 65 are down in 18 of 25 reporting countries over the period from the late 1950s to the late 1970s (see Table 7). For men under age 65, overall malignant neoplasm death rates averaged 178 per 100 000 in the late 1970s, down from 208 per 100 000 in the late 1950s. In the latest period cancer death rates of non-elderly men range from 128 per 100 000 in Sweden to 338 in Luxembourg.

Lung cancer death rates among non-elderly men average 64 deaths per 100 000 in the European region, ranging from 26 deaths per 100 000 in Portugal to 92 per

Table 6. Ischaemic heart disease; Indicator 9-2-1

Country	1957	1977	Projection
EUR	147.4	184.9	232.0
ALB	0	0	0
AUT	182.2	198.0	215.3
BEL	153.6	197.8	254.7
BUL	71.5	161.5	364.9
CZE	176.7	279.9	443.4
DDR	0	0	0
DEN	186.0	251.3	339.6
DEU	193.6	201.2	209.1
FIN	372.5	455.0	555.7
FRA	73.0	95.8	125.9
GRE	68.1	121.1	215.2
HUN	154.3	243.4	383.8
ICE	226.5	255.1	287.2
IRE	238.2	325.4	444.5
ITA	151.8	153.9	156.0
LUX	297.2	219.6	162.2
MAT	198.6	282.1	400.9
MON	0	0	0
MOR	0	0	0
NET	157.3	227.5	329.0
NOR	172.3	245.6	350.0
POL	104.9	179.2	306.3
POR	75.5	107	151.4
ROM	78.3	109.6	153.4
SMR	0	0	0
SPA	79.2	100.2	126.9
SSR	0	0	0
SWE	168.9	222.9	294.1
SWI	163.4	139.8	119.6
TUR	0	0	0
UNK	266.2	334.1	419.2
YUG	109.4	124.9	142.5

Source: WHO-Euro, Statistical Data System.
Data are age adjusted rates averaged for five years from 1955-1959 and 1975-1979. Historical data for BUL, GRE, ROM, and YUG are for 1960-1964. Historical data for LUX and MAT for 1965-1969.

100 000 in Belgium (see Table 8). Not too surprisingly, Belgium reports high cigarette consumption per capita (see Table 9).

For women under age 65, there has been little change in the cancer death rate in the 20-year period from the late 1950s to the late 1970s. The European average was 144 per 100 000 in the late 1970s compared with 146 per 100 000 in the late 1950s. In the latest period, non-elderly female cancer death rates range from 115 in Spain to 190 in Denmark (see Table 10).

Table 7. Malignant neoplasms; Indicator 10-1-1

Country	1957	1977	Projection	Target
EUR	208.1	177.6	151.5	150.9
ALB	0	0	0	0
AUT	200.7	226.2	255.0	192.3
BEL	225.6	191.3	162.2	162.6
BUL	169.0	188.3	209.9	160.1
CZE	262.6	227.7	197.5	193.6
DDR	0	0	0	0
DEN	185.1	173.9	163.3	147.8
DEU	191.1	187.9	184.7	159.7
FIN	196.5	246.4	309.0	209.4
FRA	249.0	192.9	149.4	163.9
GRE	169.8	153.2	138.1	130.2
HUN	232.3	180.9	140.9	153.7
ICE	144.9	165.4	188.8	140.6
IRE	189.6	172.6	157.1	146.7
ITA	225.0	178.0	140.9	151.3
LUX	243.0	337.6	469.0	286.9
MAT	179.2	140.7	110.4	119.6
MON	0	0	0	0
MOR	0	0	0	0
NET	202.6	181.1	161.8	153.9
NOR	145.9	142.0	138.2	120.7
POL	226.8	158.6	110.9	134.8
POR	164.1	129.4	102.0	110.0
ROM	179.9	144.9	116.7	123.2
SMR	0	0	0	0
SPA	175.8	137.2	107.0	116.6
SSR	0	0	0	0
SWE	137.4	127.9	119.1	108.7
SWI	193.3	193.6	193.8	164.5
TUR	0	0	0	0
UNK	225.8	209.9	195.1	178.4
YUG	176.7	136.4	105.3	115.9

Source: WHO-Euro Statistical Data File.
BUL, GRE, and IRE data are five year averages for 1960-1964 and 1975-1979; LUX and MAT are for 1965-1969 and 1975-1979. ROM data are ten year averages for 1950-1959 and five year for 1975-1979; all others are five year averages for 1955-1959 and 1975-1979.

Table 8. Lung cancer; Indicator 10-2-1

Country	1957	1977	Projection
EUR	46.1	64.3	89.9
ALB	0	0	0
AUT	74.1	58.2	45.7
BEL	56.6	92.1	150.0
BUL	57.9	55.0	52.2
CZE	65.8	91.0	126.0
DDR	0	0	0
DEN	43.0	61.2	86.9
DEU	52.9	57.4	62.2
FIN	83.6	81.2	78.9
FRA	32.2	55.9	97.1
GRE	38.8	55.3	78.8
HUN	40.6	68.2	114.4
ICE	25.8	33.2	42.9
IRE	43.6	62.2	88.7
ITA	35.9	72.7	147.2
LUX	122.3	90.8	67.4
MAT	48.8	67.3	92.8
MON	0	0	0
MOR	0	0	0
NET	62.7	86.5	119.3
NOR	18.3	32.7	58.4
POL	27.1	75.5	210.0
POR	12.0	26.1	56.9
ROM	30.1	53.0	93.3
SMR	0	0	0
SPA	20.7	42.0	85.2
SSR	0	0	0
SWE	19.8	27.8	39.1
SWI	48.5	66.1	90.0
TUR	0	0	0
UNK	98.3	87.4	77.7
YUG	31.1	53.2	91.1

Source: WHO-Euro Statistical Data System.
Data are age adjusted rates averaged for five years from 1955-1959 and 1975-1979. Historical data for BUL, GRE, ICE and YUG are for 1960-1964. Historical data for LUX and MAT are for 1965-1969.

Table 9. Cigarette consumption; Indicator 16-1

Country	1970	1979	Projection
EUR	2241.1	2344.3	2452.2
ALB	0	0	0
AUT	0	0	0
BEL	2945	2882	2820.3
BUL	0	0	0
CZE	0	0	0
DDR	1257	1732	2386.4
DEN	2176	2455	2769.7
DEU	2685	2843	3010.2
FIN	2252	2200	2149.2
FRA	2171	2288	2411.3
GRE	0	0	0
HUN	0	0	0
ICE	0	0	0
IRE	3015	3381	3791.4
ITA	2093	2643	3337.5
LUX	0	0	0
MAT	0	0	0
MON	0	0	0
MOR	0	0	0
NET	2963	3508	4153.2
NOR	2074	1995	1919.0
POL	0	0	0
POR	0	0	0
ROM	0	0	0
SMR	0	0	0
SPA	0	0	0
SSR	1970	1980	1990.0
SWE	0	0	0
SWI	0	0	0
TUR	0	0	0
UNK	3244	3070	2905.3
YUG	0	0	0

Source: Various Country Reports.

Table 10. Malignant neoplasms; Indicator 10-1-2

Country	1957	1977	Projection	Target
EUR	145.9	143.6	141.4	122.1
ALB	0	0	0	0
AUT	179.8	156.0	135.4	132.6
BEL	164.7	152.5	141.2	129.6
BUL	124.9	118.2	111.8	100.4
CZE	167.3	157.7	148.7	134.1
DDR	0	0	0	0
DEN	188.8	190.3	191.8	161.8
DEU	169.7	154.4	140.4	131.2
FIN	148.6	120.4	97.5	102.3
FRA	139.4	127.0	115.6	107.9
GRE	109.4	116.2	123.4	98.7
HUN	166.9	171.0	175.2	145.3
ICE	175.8	153.2	133.4	130.2
IRE	170.3	179.3	188.8	152.4
ITA	139.9	136.6	133.3	116.1
LUX	207.0	153.7	114.2	130.7
MAT	95.2	114.5	137.5	97.3
MON	0	0	0	0
MOR	0	0	0	0
NET	158.7	148.0	138.1	125.8
NOR	148.6	139.5	131.0	118.6
POL	135.4	150.4	167.0	127.8
POR	116.7	119.1	121.7	101.3
ROM	130.4	135.4	140.6	115.1
SMR	0	0	0	0
SPA	112.2	114.6	117.0	97.4
SSR	0	0	0	0
SWE	151.4	141.1	131.5	119.9
SWI	154.1	135.0	118.3	114.7
TUR	0	0	0	0
UNK	166.7	180.5	195.5	153.4
YUG	116.1	120.5	125.1	102.4

Source: WHO-Euro Statistical Data File.
BUL, GRE, and IRE data are five year averages for 1960-1964 and 1975-1979; LUX and MAT are for 1965-1969 and 1975-1979; Rom data are ten year averages for 1950-1959 and five year for 1975-1979; others are five year averages for 1955-1959 and 1975-1979.

Breast cancer death rates of women under age 65 average 34 deaths per 100 000 in the European region, ranging from 22 deaths per 100 000 in Romania to 51 per 100 000 in the United Kingdom (see Table 11). Cervical cancer death rates of non-elderly women average 8 per 100 000 in the European region, but range from 2 per 100 000 in Italy and Spain to 18 in Poland and 19 in Romania (see Table 12).

No clear picture emerges from these variations in cancer death rates by cause and age-sex group. However, substantial variations do occur. Data on these rates could be extremely helpful to researchers and public health officials wishing to pinpoint and combat major health problems.

Alcohol Consumption

A WHO-EURO report by Walsh [5] presents information on alcohol consumption in many of the European member states. In 1979, European countries included in the study averaged 14.6 l alcohol per person aged 15 and over (see Table 13). France had the highest average at 20.5 l, followed by Portugal and Spain at 19.6 l. Norway at 5.7 l and Sweden at 7.6 l per capita were at the low end of the range.

Liver cirrhosis death rates for men ages 65 to 84 averaged 120 per 100 000 for Europe as a whole in the late 1970s (see Table 14). Death rates from this cause, however, ranged from 6.8 in Iceland (which did not report data on alcohol consumption in the Walsh study) to 214 per 100 000 in Italy. Portugal had a liver cirrhosis death rate of 203 per 100 000, Spain 151 per 100 000, and France 183 per 100 000 – all considerably above the European average. Low alcohol consumption countries such as Norway averaged a liver cirrhosis death rate of elderly males of 21 per 100 000 and Sweden of 42 per 100 000, considerably below the European average.

Health and the Elderly

Measures of disability, functioning, and prevalence of chronic conditions will be added to the WHO-EURO health indicator data base in the future. At present, the best measure of overall health status available in the health indicator data base is life expectancy of men and women at age 65. This measure captures the expected longevity of those who survive to old age.

Men in the European region reaching age 65 in 1980 can expect to live on to age 78, on average (see Table 15). However, this ranges from age 81 in Iceland to 76 in Malta and 77 in Hungary and Czechoslovakia.

Women reaching age 65 in 1980 can expect to live on to age 82, on average, substantially above the life expectancy for men (see Table 16). Iceland also has the highest life expectancy for women at age 65. Women living to age 65 can expect to live on to age 85 in Iceland, compared with age 80 in Malta, and 81 in Romania.

Table 11. Breast cancer; Indicator 10-3-3

Country	1957	1977	Projection
EUR	24.7	34.0	46.9
ALB	0	0	0
AUT	26.3	34.2	44.5
BEL	35.3	44.0	54.9
BUL	19.8	25.5	32.8
CZE	22.6	31.5	43.7
DDR	0	0	0
DEN	39.4	46.0	53.7
DEU	27.7	36.4	47.9
FIN	24.8	26.7	28.7
FRA	26.3	32.6	40.3
GRE	13.1	26.1	52.0
HUN	22.0	34.8	55.1
ICE	49.2	38.8	30.7
IRE	37.6	48.2	61.6
ITA	25.6	34.5	46.4
LUX	43	40.8	38.7
MAT	28	38.4	52.7
MON	0	0	0
MOR	0	0	0
NET	40.2	45.3	51.1
NOR	31.1	32.2	33.3
POL	10.2	26.6	69.2
POR	19.4	26.8	36.9
ROM	9.2	22.4	54.3
SMR	0	0	0
SPA	11.3	25.6	57.5
SSR	0	0	0
SWE	32.7	31.4	30.1
SWI	36.8	40.9	45.4
TUR	0	0	0
UNK	41.4	50.8	62.3
YUG	14.2	22.6	36.0

Source: WHO-Euro Statistical Data System.
Data are age adjusted rates averaged for five years from 1955-1959 and 1975-1979. Historical data BUL, GRE, ICE, and YUG are for 1960-1964. Historical data for LUX and MAT are for 1965-1969.

Table 12. Cancer cervix uteri; Indicator 10-3-1

Country	1957	1977	Projection
EUR	8.2	8.3	8.5
ALB	0	0	0
AUT	6.8	8.9	11.6
BEL	9.1	5.4	3.2
BUL	4.8	5.4	6.1
CZE	13.4	9.7	7.0
DDR	0	0	0
DEN	22.9	17.2	13.0
DEU	7.9	9.6	11.7
FIN	10.8	4.8	2.1
FRA	6	4.7	3.7
GRE	0.9	2.3	5.9
HUN	5.9	12.2	25.0
ICE	11.9	8.7	6.3
IRE	5.3	6.0	6.9
ITA	3.8	1.9	1.0
LUX	20.9	7.8	2.9
MAT	5.2	5.3	5.5
MON	0	0	0
MOR	0	0	0
NET	12.7	7.9	4.9
NOR	15.3	10.9	7.7
POL	7.2	17.5	42.1
POR	18.7	8.6	3.9
ROM	14.1	19.4	26.8
SMR	0	0	0
SPA	0.6	1.9	6.0
SSR	0	0	0
SWE	9.8	7.3	5.4
SWI	14.3	8.0	4.5
TUR	0	0	0
UNK	13.7	11.4	9.5
YUG	7.7	8.8	10.0

Source: WHO-Euro Statistical Data System.
Data are age adjusted rates averaged for five years from 1955-1959 and 1975-1979. Historical data for BUL, GRE, ICE, and YUG are for 1960-1964. Historical data for LUX and MAT are for 1965-1969.

Table 13. Alcohol consumption; Indicator 17-1

Country	1950	1979	Projection
EUR	8.5	14.6	25.2
ALB	0	0	0
AUT	6.5	14.3	31.4
BEL	8	14.4	25.9
BUL	0	0	0
CZE	5.3	13.5	34.3
DDR	1.6	10.6	70.2
DEN	4.9	12.2	30.3
DEU	3.8	16	67.3
FIN	2.4	8.1	27.3
FRA	22.1	20.5	19.0
GRE	0	0	0
HUN	6.4	15.7	38.5
ICE	0	0	0
IRE	4.6	11.3	27.7
ITA	12.4	16.1	20.9
LUX	8.5	16.8	33.2
MAT	0	0	0
MON	0	0	0
MOR	0	0	0
NET	3	12.2	49.6
NOR	2.9	5.7	11.2
POL	4.3	10.8	27.1
POR	0	19.6	0
ROM	0	0	0
SMR	0	0	0
SPA	0	19.6	0
SSR	0	0	0
SWE	4.7	7.6	12.2
SWI	10.4	13.5	17.5
TUR	0	0	0
UNK	6.3	10.3	16.8
YUG	0	12	0

Source: D. Walsh, Alcohol-related medicosocial problems and their prevention. WHO-Euro, Copenhagen, 1982, p. 21.

Table 14. Liver cirrhosis; Indicator 17-5-3

Country	1957	1977	Projection
EUR	79.5	119.5	179.4
ALB	0	0	0
AUT	129.4	183.6	260.5
BEL	52.2	73.6	103.8
BUL	36.5	51.0	71.3
CZE	56.2	97.8	169.9
DDR	0	0	0
DEN	32.4	35.2	38.2
DEU	105.2	148.1	208.3
FIN	22.4	23.0	23.6
FRA	147.9	182.7	225.7
GRE	114.2	88.3	68.2
HUN	52.1	107.2	220.5
ICE	23.8	6.8	1.9
IRE	9.0	14.8	24.2
ITA	117.4	214.2	391.1
LUX	172.0	151.7	133.7
MAT	65.6	95.0	137.7
MON	0	0	0
MOR	0	0	0
NET	23.7	26.4	29.5
NOR	18.4	20.8	23.5
POL	19.9	85.0	362.0
POR	170.9	202.6	240.1
ROM	0	0	0
SMR	0	0	0
SPA	100.6	151.0	226.5
SSR	0	0	0
SWE	23.5	41.9	74.7
SWI	115.9	96.0	79.4
TURb	0	0	0
UNK	12.7	14.8	17.3
YUG	52.1	104.5	209.6

Source: WHO-Euro Statistical Data System.
Data are age adjusted rates averaged for five years from 1955-1959 and 1975-1979. Historical data for BUL, GRE, ICE, and YUG are for 1960-1964. Historical data for LUX and MAT are for 1965-1969.

Table 15. Life expectancy males; Indicator 6-2-5

Country	1960	1980	Projection
EUR	13.1	13.2	13.2
ALB	14.7	0	0
AUT	12.1	13	13.9
BEL	12.4	12.8	13.2
BUL	13.5	12.6	11.7
CZE	12.3	11.7	11.1
DDR	12.7	12.1	11.5
DEN	13.8	13.7	13.6
DEU	12.3	13	13.7
FIN	11.5	12.5	13.5
FRA	12.5	14.1	15.9
GRE	13.5	15.5	17.7
HUN	12	11.6	11.2
ICE	15	15.8	16.6
IRE	12	12.4	12.8
ITA	13.4	13.8	14.2
LUX	0	12.6	0
MAT	11.8	11.2	10.6
MON	0	0	0
MOR	0	0	0
NET	14.1	14	13.9
NOR	14.6	14.4	14.2
POL	12.6	12.2	11.8
POR	12.4	12.2	12.0
ROM	12.1	12.5	12.9
SMR	0	0	0
SPA	12.8	14.1	15.5
SSR	14	0	0
SWE	13.9	14.4	14.9
SWI	0	14.4	0
TUR	0	0	0
UNK	12.1	12.8	13.5
YUG	12.1	13.1	14.1

Source: WHO, World Health Statistics Annual.

Table 16. Life expectancy females; Indicator 6-2-6

Country	1960	1980	Projection
EUR	15.5	16.6	17.8
ALB	16.8	0	0
AUT	14.8	16.4	18.1
BEL	14.8	16.6	18.6
BUL	14.7	14.7	14.7
CZE	14.5	14.9	15.3
DDR	14.6	14.8	15.0
DEN	15.1	17.8	20.9
DEU	14.5	16.8	19.4
FIN	13.7	16.8	20.6
FRA	15.6	18.5	21.9
GRE	15.1	17.5	20.2
HUN	13.6	14.7	15.8
ICE	16.8	19.5	22.6
IRE	14.4	15.5	16.6
ITA	15.3	17.3	19.5
LUX	0	16	0
MAT	13.4	13.1	12.8
MON	0	0	0
MOR	0	0	0
NET	15.4	18.7	22.7
NOR	16	18.3	20.9
POL	14.8	15.7	16.6
POR	14.6	15.2	15.8
ROM	13.4	14.2	15.0
SMR	0	0	0
SPA	14.8	17.1	19.7
SSR	16.8	0	0
SWE	15.2	18.2	21.7
SWI	0	18.4	0
TUR	0	0	0
UNK	15.2	16.9	18.7
YUG	13.8	15.3	16.9

Source: WHO, World Health Statistics Annual.

Potential Uses of a Health Indicator Reporting System

These preliminary results should be viewed with considerable caution. Countries vary in the accuracy of reporting even death rate information [4] . Data on life-styles, such as alcohol and smoking behavior may be even less accurate. However, many of the broad patterns presented here are likely to persist even as data collection and reporting practices become more standardized. The central message is that health outcomes vary markedly even among countries with high levels of economic, scientific, and educational development. Further, it seems unlikely that this variation is totally random, but undoubtedly is linked to lifestyle and environmental health risks, socioeconomic factors, preventive health measures, and the distribution and content of health care.

Establishment of a health indicator data base should prove helpful in several regards. First, it can help focus attention of policy officials and researchers on major problem areas. Knowing a problem exists, and some indication of its magnitude and the historical direction of change, is clearly a first step for generating appropriate action.

Second, information on a number of health indicators may be helpful in establishing resource allocation priorities. Countries for which accidental death rates are a particularly serious problem may decide to concentrate more resources in that area, while countries for which heart disease death rates are a particularly serious problem may wish to direct more attention to those factors contributing to heart disease. Given budgetary pressures common to many countries, information to guide budgetary priorities can be extremely critical. An indicator-based system can also provide an early warning system by detecting when budget cutbacks are having a deleterious effect on health [1] .

Third, comparable information on a number of countries may point to successful strategies for improving health. Experiences of countries with relatively good performance on some measures can be explored, with a view to identifying contributing causes.

Finally, the existence of a rich health indicator data base facilitates systematic empirical research on the determinants of health outcomes. As additional data are added to the health targets indicator data base and as accuracy and standardization of definitions on a wide range of indicators are attained, researchers will find this a fruitful area for investigation. It should foster interdisciplinary research drawing on the talents of investigators with backgrounds in epidemiology, health services research, behavioral science, economics, and medicine, among others. Out of this activity should come greater insight and advances which should advance the overall goal of assuring health for all people.

References

1. R.J. Blendon and D.E. Rogers, "Cutting Medical Care Costs: Primum Non Nocere", Journal of the American Medical Association, Vol. 250, No. 14 (October 14, 1983), pp. 1880-1885

2. Z. Brzezinski, Regional Targets in Support of the Regional Strategy for Health for All, Epidemiological Background. Regional Committee for Europe, World Health Organization, Document EUR/RC34/5, 1984

3. K. Davis, European Regional Targets Project: Microcomputer Software Package. Document prepared for the World Health Organization, European Regional Office, October 1, 1984

4. International Journal of Epidemiology, Editorial "Improving Data Bases for International Studies", Vol. 13, No.3, 1984, pp. 267-268

5. D. Walsh, Alcohol-Related Medicosocial Problems and their Prevention. World Health Organization, European Regional Office, 1982

6. World Health Organization, World Health Assembly Resolution WHA 30.43, 1977

7. World Health Organization, European Regional Office, Regional Committee Document EUR/RC30/8 Rev.2, 1980

8. World Health Organization, European Regional Office, Regional Targets in Support of the Regional Strategy for Health for All. Regional Committee Document EUR/RC34/7, 1984

9. World Health Organization, European Regional Office, List of Proposed Indicatores for Monitoring Progress Toward Health for All in the European Region. Regional Committee Document EUR/RC34/13, 1984

Appendix A: European Countries in Microcomputer Data System

1.	EUR	Europe
2.	ALB	Albania
3.	AUT	Austria
4.	BEL	Belgium
5.	BUL	Bulgaria
6.	CZE	Czechoslovakia
7.	DDR	German Democratic Republic
8.	DEN	Denmark
9.	DEU	Federal Republic of Germany
10.	FIN	Finland
11.	FRA	France
12.	GRE	Greece
13.	HUN	Hungary
14.	ICE	Iceland
15.	IRE	Ireland
16.	ITA	Italy
17.	LUX	Luxembourg
18.	MAT	Malta
19.	MON	Monaco
20.	MOR	Morroco
21.	NET	Netherlands
22.	NOR	Norway
23.	POL	Poland
24.	POR	Portugal
25.	ROM	Romania
26.	SMR	San Marino
27.	SPA	Spain
28.	SSR	U. S. S. R.
29.	SWE	Sweden
30.	SWI	Switzerland
31.	TUR	Turkey
32.	UNK	United Kingdom
33.	YUG	Yugoslavia

Appendix B: European Regional Targets

1. Reducing Inequalities*
2. Promoting Health*
3. Opportunity for Disabled*
4. Reducing Disease
5. Elimination of Disease
6. Life Expectancy
7. Infant Mortality
8. Maternal Mortality
9. Heart Disease
10. Cancer
11. Accidents
12. Suicide
13. Healthy Public Policy*
14. Social Support*
15. Health Education
16. Healthy Behaviour
17. Damaging Behaviour
18. Environmental Health*
19. Environmental Risks*
20. Water Pollution
21. Air Pollution*
22. Food Safety
23. Hazardous Waste*
24. Housing*
25. Working Environment*
26. Primary Health Care
27. Resource Distribution
28. Primary Health Care Content
29. Primary Health Care Providers*
30. Resource Coordination*
31. Quality*
32. Research*
33. Health Policy*
34. Planning
35. Health Information*
36. Health Personnel*
37. Health Education*
38. Health Technology*

---

* Indicates targets with no indicator data currently in system.

Appendix C: European Regional Target Indicators. Data Currently in Microcomputer Data System

Target 4 Reducing disease and disablement

4. 3. 1 Cases of tuberculosis per 100000 population
4. 3. 2 Cases of intestinal infectious diseases per 100000
4. 3. 3 Cases of hepatitis per 100000
4. 3. 4 Cases of veneral disease per 100000
4. 3. 5 Cases of influenza per 100000

Target 5 Elimination of diseases

5. 1. 1 Cases of measles per 100000
5. 1. 2 Cases of malaria per 100000

Target 6 Life Expectancy

6. 1. 1 Life expectancy at birth males
6. 1. 2 Life expectancy at birth females
6. 2. 1 Life expectancy at age 15 males
6. 2. 2 Life expectancy at age 15 females
6. 2. 3 Life expectancy at age 45 males
6. 2. 4 Life expectancy at age 45 females
6. 2. 5 Life expectancy at age 65 males
6. 2. 6 Life expectancy at age 65 females

Target 7 Infant mortality

7. 1 Infant mortality rate
7. 2 Neonatal mortality rate
7. 3 Postneonatal mortality rate
7. 4 Perinatal mortality rate

Target 8 Maternal mortality

8. 1 Maternal mortality rate

Target 9 Heart disease

9. 2. 1 Ischaemic heart death rate males 35-64
9. 2. 2 Ischaemic heart death rate females 35-64
9. 2. 3 Ischaemic heart death rate males 65-84
9. 2. 4 Ischaemic heart death rate females 65-84
9. 3. 1 Cerebrovascular death rate males 35-64
9. 3. 2 Cerebrovascular death rate females 35-64
9. 3. 3 Cerebrovascular death rate males 65-84
9. 3. 4 Cerebrovascular death rate females 65-84

Target 10	Cancer
10. 1. 1	Malignant neoplasm death rate males 30-64
10. 1. 2	Malignant neoplasm death rate females 30-64
10. 1. 3	Malignant neoplasm death rate males 65-84
10. 1. 4	Malignant neoplasm death rate females 65-84
10. 2. 1	Lung cancer death rate males 30-64
10. 2. 2	Lung cancer death rate females 30-64
10. 2. 3	Lung cancer death rate males 65-84
10. 2. 4	Lung cancer death rate females 65-84
10. 3. 1	Cancer of cervix uteri 30-64
10. 3. 2	Cancer of cervix uteri 65-84
10. 3. 3	Breast cancer death rate 30-64
10. 3. 4	Breast cancer death rate 65-84
10. 4. 1	New cases of cancer per 100000 M
10. 4. 2	New cases of cancer per 100000 F
Target 11	Accidents
11. 1. 1	External causes death rate males 5-64
11. 1. 2	External causes death rate females 5-64
11. 1. 3	External causes death rate males 65-84
11. 1. 4	External causes death rate females 65-84
11. 2. 1	Motor vehicle traffic accident death rate males 5-64
11. 2. 2	Motor vehicle traffic accident death rate females 5-64
11. 2. 3	Motor vehicle traffic accident death rate males 65-84
11. 2. 4	Motor vehicle traffic accident death rate females 65-84
Target 12	Suicide
12. 1. 1	Suicide death rate males 10-64
12. 1. 2	Suicide death rate females 10-64
12. 1. 3	Suicide death rate males 65-84
12. 1. 4	Suicide death rate females 65-84
Target 15	Education for health
15. 2. 1	Adult literacy rate total
15. 2. 2	Adult literacy rate males
15. 2. 3	Adult literacy rate females
Target 16	Promoting healthy behaviour
16. 1	Cigarette consumption per capita
16. 3. 1	Food supply of calories per capita
16. 3. 2	Food supply of protein per capita
16. 3. 3	Food supply of fat per capita
16. 4	Low birth weight infants

Target 17	Reducing damaging behaviour
17. 1	Alcohol consumption per capita in liters
17. 3. 1	Consumption of cocaine per 1000000
17. 3. 2	Consumption of codeine per 1000000
17. 3. 3	Consumption of dextropropoxyphene per 1000000
17. 3. 4	Consumption of dihydrocodeine per 1000000
17. 3. 5	Consumption of diphenoxylate per 1000000
17. 3. 6	Consumption of ethylmorphine per 1000000
17. 3. 7	Consumption of methadone per 1000000
17. 3. 8	Consumption of morphine per 1000000
17. 3. 9	Consumption of oxycodone per 1000000
17. 3. 10	Consumption of pethidine per 1000000
17. 3. 11	Consumption of pholcodine per 1000000
17. 5. 1	Liver cirrhosis death rate males 30-64
17. 5. 2	Liver cirrhosis death rate females 30-64
17. 5. 3	Liver cirrhosis death rate males 65-84
17. 5. 4	Liver cirrhosis death rate females 65-84
17. 6	Consumption of psychotropic substances per capita

Target 20	Water pollution
20. 1. 1	Percent population served by piped public water supply
20. 1. 2	Percent population served by sewerage systems

Target 22	Food safety
22. 2	Food poisoning cases per capita

Target 27	Distribution of resources
27. 1	Percent of national health expenditures devoted to local care
27. 2. 1	Physisians per 100000
27. 2. 2	Nurses per 100000
27. 2. 3	Dentists per 100000
27. 2. 4	Pharmacists per 100000
27. 2. 5	Hospital beds per 100000
27. 2. 6	Hospital admissions per 100000
27. 2. 7	Hospital occupancy rates

Target 28	Primary health care
28. 1. 1	Percent of infants immunized for DPT
28. 1. 2	Percent of infants immunized for measles
28. 1. 3	Percent of infants immunized for polio
28. 1. 4	Percent of infants immunized for TB
28. 2. 1	Birth rate

28. 2. 2	Fertility rate
28. 5	Abortions per 1000 births
Target 34	Planning and resource allocation
34. 1	Percent of GNP spent on health

9/18/84

Trends in Health and Health Care

5. Demographic Indicator Systems of Health Care Needs

Gail Wilensky and Steven Chapman

Concern over inflation in the health care sector must, if it is to lead to useful commentary, address itself to the factors that influence the level of health care expenditures. Observers whose concerns are to contain costs as painlessly as possible tend to focus on factors that are products of particular policy choice. Presumably, the intention is to select the policy option or options which could cut "fat" from the systems, thereby lowering expenditures without adversely affecting quality and which would promote efficiency in the delivery of health care. This focus is wholly appropriate; policy makers should be aware of all of the tools at their disposal to shape and develop the health care system, and what effects their past use of these tools has had. They should know of the effects of various reimbursement systems, and of different strategies for capital investment in new technologies. Familiarity with these factors leads to a broader understanding of the alternatives open to policy makers, and, quite possibly, more insightful policy.

It is also important for policy makers to gauge the environment within which any policy choice must be made. Part of the environment that has, and will, change is reflected in demographics. This paper is an examination of the role of changing demographics, and of indicator systems that will help us monitor future changes in that role.

There are factors other than demographics that influence the level of health care expenditures, but that are not so clearly a product of a particular policy choice. Societal norms, for example, do not always dictate policy, but they do roughly delineate boundaries within which policy is kept. These norms address the "proper" amount of responsibility to the ill, aged, and aged ill, as well as whether that responsibility should be borne by the federal, state, or local government, private organizations, or families. Norms can change swiftly, as we have witnessed in the emergence of the welfare state in this century. The shape that these societal norms acquire in the future will be an important factor to the level of health care expenditures. Policy makers can, under certain circumstances, influence these norms but in the final analysis, it is the norm that must justify the policy, not the policy that must justify the norm.

The status and strength of a nation's economy will also affect the level of spending on health. While policy makers can significantly influence the course of the economy, they cannot control it completely. Furthermore, the effects of economic policies are frequently long term and difficult to predict. If an economy falters, and slips into a deep and prolonged recession, the total amount of health care expenditures is likely to decline. In general, countries with a higher gross national product

(GNP) spend more on health although the percentage of GNP spent on health reflects many factors other than just the wealth of the country. Another set of factors that influence the level of health care expenditures which is even further out of the hands of policy makers is demographics. If the mortality rates of a given society go down, if morbidity rates go up and if all other factors remain unchanged, then the amount spent on health will almost certainly rise. Factors such as these that affect health care expenditure rates, but are not directly controlled by policy-makers are nonetheless important for policy-makers to understand. They can increase pressure on policy-makers and stress throughout the health system if they increase expenditures, and decrease pressure on policy makers and stress throughout the system if they decrease expenditures.

This paper examines the effects of demographic changes on health care expenditures in the past, and possible effects in the future. Although in any given year not much change and therefore not much effect is found - especially in relation to the change in and effect of other factors such as hospital inputs cost inflation - a demographic trend that holds for several years may indeed significantly impact health care spending and force policy makers to reassess certain programmes and delivery systems.

Demographic Trends

It is no secret that developed nations are experiencing unprecedented growth in the size of their elderly (65 and over) population, and even greater growth in the size of the very elderly (85 and over) population. Due to a combination of lifestyle, nutritional, environmental and medical factors, the average life expectancy for a US citizen at birth has risen from 47.3 years in 1900 to 74.5 in 1982 [1] , and the elderly population has nearly tripled as a percentage of total population [2] . Within this growing segment of the population, there are certain subgroups that have been growing even faster.

For example, since 1950, the number of people who are 85 or older has grown twice as fast as those who are 65 or older [2] . Over the same time span, the minority elderly population has also grown at twice the rate of the white elderly population, and the female elderly population has grown at about 1 1/2 times the rate of the elderly male population [3] .

These trends are expected by the general consensus of observers to continue - although there remains room for disagreement over how large future increases will actually be. This is exemplified by the Census Bureau's 1972 underestimation by 6.6% of what the size of the elderly population would be in 1980 [4] . This error was due to an unpredicted decline in mortality, and was characteristic of the Census Bureau's tendency throughout the 1960s and 1970s to underestimate mortality rates. A response to these inaccuracies led by demographers Kenneth G. Manton, Eileen M. Crimmins, and Barbara B. Torrey contends that mortality rates will continue to fall, and that the Census continues to underestimate the future size of the elderly population. The response argument seems to be winning the debate. The Census projections of May, 1984 include much lower mortality assumptions than their previous projections, although not quite as low as Manton's, Crimmins', and Torrey's assumptions. Besides reluctance within the Census to so drastically alter their mortality assumptions, this probably is due to the greater importance attached by the Census to the deceleration in the decline of mortality rates since the late 1970s. Yet even though differences between these two groups over the rate of growth of the elderly population remain, there is mutual agreement that it will grow and be a factor to be reckoned with for policy-makers.

According to the Census, the percentage of the population which is 65 or older is expected to rise from 12.0 in 1985 to 13.0 in 2000. The percentage 85 or older will rise from 1.1 to 1.8 in the year 2000 meaning that not only is the general population aging, but the "very old" population is increasing at a disproportionately faster rate. In fact, in absolute numbers, the total number of people 65-69 years old will increase by only 157 965 between 1982 and 2000, whereas the total number of people 85-89 years old will increase by 1 693 314 [2] .

The problems posed by this increase in the elderly population are exacerbated by a decrease in the growth rate of the total population. Overall growth in the US population was 18.6% between 1950-1960, 11.0% between 1970-1980, and is expected by the Census to be 7.3% between 1990-2000 [2] . If the retirement age remains 65, the aged support ratio (the number of people aged 65 and over divided by the number of people in the "working population" aged 18-64) would rise from 0.1859 in 1980 to 0.2116 in 2000, an increase of 13.8% percent [2] . This ratio reflects the number of potential beneficiaries of health insurance programmes in relation to wage earners, who will pay for many of the programmes.

When the "baby-boom" generation becomes elderly around 2030, there will be a large and rapid increase in the elderly population. Between 2010 and 2030, the 65 and over population will increase from 13.8% to 21.2% of the total population and rise in absolute numbers from 392 million to 64.6 million. Between 2030 and 2050, the 85 and over population will increase from 2.8% to 5.2% of the total population, and rise in absolute numbers from 8.6 million to 16.0 million [2] .

Mortality rates in the US remained relatively constant between 1954 and 1968, declined from the late 1960s to late 1970s, and have leveled off into the early 1980s. There are no unmistakable indicators of what future mortality trends will be, but, if they remain at current rates of decline, there will be increasing utilization levels of health care.

Health Care Utilization

The elderly already have relatively high health care utilization rates. This follows reasonably from the fact that the health status of the elderly is generally poorer than that of the non-elderly. At the present, the elderly have relatively high morbidity rates: 85% have at least one chronic condition (with an average of four chronic conditions among this 85% [5]), and acute conditions are associated with twice as many days of restricted activity for the elderly as they are for the non-elderly. Forty-six percent of the elderly suffer from a disabling illness, contrasted with 7.3% of those 45 and under and 24.1% of those 46-64 [6].

Health care utilization rates for the elderly reflect their generally poorer health status. Despite composing only 11% of the population in 1980, the elderly accounted for 38% of all hospitals days, 15% of all physician visits, 87% of all nursing home residents, and 29% of all personal health care expenditures. Assuming that the Census Bureau's mortality rate projections are accurate or low and that current utilization rates continue, there will be a substantial increase in the size of the health sector over the next few decades. Between 1980 and 2040, the percentage of all physician visits made by the elderly will increase from 15 to 27, the increase in total hospital care will be even greater, because age-specific utilization rates for hospital care vary more than those for physician visits. The percentage of all short-stay hospital days accumulated by the elderly will increase from 38 to 57 by 2040. The amount of nursing home care will rise even faster. The number of residents, most of whom are elderly, will more than triple by 2040 and increase from 9.4% to 13% of total personal health care expenditures. Such increasing utilization rates will lead to higher expenditures: the percentage of total personal health care expenditures spent by the elderly will rise from 29 to 45 over the same period.

Increases of this nature and magnitude would undoubtedly force a reassessment of the health care system followed by decisions on how much we want our society to spend on health care. For now, however, it is our task to evaluate the preceding projections, postulate alternative developments, and finally discuss indicators that could be monitored to see what demographic trends actually emerge.

Trends in Mortality and Morbidity

Uncertainty that could jeopardize the preceding projections is found in mortality, morbidity, and disability rate assumptions. The first, mortality rates, have already proven difficult to predict, as discussed earlier. Still, observers who recognize this difficulty disagree only over how fast they will decline, not whether they will decline or not. It seems that, barring an unanticipated drastic change in environment, lifestyle, nutritional, or medical factors, mortality rates will continue to fall.

Morbidity and disability rate assumptions are the focus of more heated controversy, and are more difficult to assess than mortality rate assumptions. James Fries argues, in his "compression of morbidity" thesis, that the health problems of our society more and more involve chronic rather than acute conditions and that the onset of these chronic conditions is delayed and the severity lessened. Therefore, he concludes, although the maximum lifespan will not increase much more, morbidity rates will fall. His is one of the more optimistic outlooks on changing demographics for, if he is right, not only will the quality of elderly life be higher than anticipated by most, but health care utilization rates and costs will be lower [7].

A conflicting theory is proposed by M. Kramer and E.M. Gruenberg [8]. They believe that the onset of chronic conditions will not appreciably change, but that fewer people will die from these chronic conditions. This outlook is decidedly more pessimistic than Fries's; people will live longer, but they will have more chronic illnesses for longer periods of time which will both lower the quality of their lives and increase the costs of their health care.

Disability rates are related to, but not the same as, morbidity rates. A chronic condition may exist in an individual, while he/she may not suffer any disability. If Kramer and Gruenberg are right about increasing chronic illness incidences, but treatment techniques improve such that a chronic illness does not cause as much disability as it currently does, then the health needs of the elderly may not increase as much as they predict.

We need to know what mortality, morbidity and disability rates are doing so that policy makers know how the health needs of the elderly are changing. It is therefore necessary to have some way of monitoring these demographic measures.

The most readily available indicators are based on cross-sectional data projected into the future. This technique is well illustrated by the efforts of Rice and Feldman discussed earlier. There are serious potential problems with this method, however; it necessitates the assumption that current demographic rates will not change. If, for example, declining mortality rates were a result of either delayed onset or the slower progression of chronic illnesses, the unqualified projection of current morbidity rates would overestimate future health care needs. Because changes in demographic rates are important and difficult to predict, cross-sectional data provide inadequate indicators; longitudinal studies are also necessary.

Mortality data that show time trends are currently in much greater abundance than are morbidity data that show time trends. These data could give some insight into morbidity trends in that underlying and associated causes of death are usually recorded, so it is possible to find out which and what type of illnesses cause death at various ages and which and what type of illnesses are present at death at various ages.

Some observers have suggested that close scrutiny of these mortality data can serve as a reasonable proxy not only for morbidity rates, but disability and health care utilization rates too. Victor Fuchs argues that measuring proximity to death rather than age may be a more accurate predictor of the future health needs of the elderly than projections based on current cross-sectional data. His rationale is that the highest concentration of medical expenditure occurs within the 3 years prior to death. Thus the proximity to death would be a more accurate prediction than chronological age. Implicit in Fuchs' reasoning is the assumption that while mortality rates fall and people live longer lives, morbidity and disability rates hold relatively steady. Insofar as the relationship between mortality and disability is variable, however, this indicator will yield an inaccurate image of the health needs of the elderly.

There is conflicting evidence to date on the patterns of morbidity and disability rates. An analysis of the National Health Survey indicates that although acute-condition incidence rates have dropped slightly since 1957, restricted activity and bed disability for them have increased [9] . Chronic conditions, on the other hand, have increased both in prevalence and limitations, which combines with the changes in acute conditions to account for a rise in total restricted activity stemming from any source among middle aged and older people.

If we are going to primarily rely on national mortality data as the basis of indicators, we will need to develop analytical models which can incorporate other measures of health status provided by clinical and community studies. Specifically, epidemiological data will be needed on the distribution of age at onset of disease and the distribution of time spent with chronic disease. These data used in conjunction with stochastic compartment models will permit the inference of changes in morbidity from changes in mortality and thus the future medical need for health service.

Outlook

The most direct measures of indicators, however, would require the development of a longitudinal data base. Only in this way will we clearly be able to observe changes in onset rates and progression rates of chronic diseases, the distribution of different chronic diseases across subpopulations and across time and changes in the distribution and incidence of acute condition desires over time. These data, used with updated estimates of population changes, would provide medically related demands for medical care. The latter, used in conjunction with alternative financing mechanisms, societal norms, and production and delivery patterns, would form the basis of future projections of health care resources and expenditure outcomes.

References

1. National Center for Health Statistics: Health, United States, 1983, DHHS Pub. No. (PHS) 84-1232, 1983

2. Bureau of the Census: Projections of the Population of the United States by Age, Sex, and Race, 1983 to 2080

3. Bureau of the Census: Statistical Abstract of the United States: 1982-83 (103 rd edition) Washington, D.C., 1982

4. Manton, K.G.: Changing Concepts of Morbidity and Mortality in the Elderly Population. Milbank Memorial Fund Quarterly 60 (2): 229-230, 1982

5. Commission on Chronic Illness

6. Rice, D.P., Feldman, J.J.: Living Longer in the United States: Demographic Changes and Health Needs of the Elderly. Milbank Memorial Fund Quarterly 61 (3): 364, 1983

7. Fries, J.: Aging, Natural Death and the Compression of Morbidity. New England Journal of Medicine 303: 130-135, 1980

8. Gruenberg, E.M.: The Failures of Success. Milbank Memorial Fund Quarterly 55 (1): 3-24, 1977

9. Verbrugge, L.M.: Longer Life But Worsening Health? Trends in Health and Mortality of Middle-Aged and Older Persons. Milbank Memorial Fund Quarterly 62 (3), 1984

6. Comments on the Paper "Demographic Indicator Systems of Health Care Needs"

Elisabeth Schach

G. Wilensky's and S. Chapman's paper examines the effects of demographic changes in population structure on health care expenditures in the past and their possible effects in the future. Due to the fact that the elderly portion of the population is expected to increase between now and the end of the century and beyond, they foresee a higher than proportional increase in health expenditures up to 2040, when it is predicted that the percentage of personal health care expenditures spent on the elderly will have risen to over 45% of total health care expenditures for the USA. They then critically review some of the assumptions of the stated predictions and suggest the development of long-term monitoring systems in order to describe long-term demographic trends, symptoms and diseases in a population as a basis for allocating health care resources in the future.

These comments relate to three aspects of the paper, namely:

1. The effect of mortality rate decreases on health care expenditures
2. The relationship between the reduction of mortality and the concurrent trend in morbidity
3. The distribution of health services use

Effect of Mortality Rate Decreases on Health Care Expenditures

The proportion of the population over the age of 65 years has been increasing due to falling mortality rates and it is predicted that it will continue to grow in years to come. One projection for the Federal Republic of Germany indicates it to be 15.2% of the total FRG population in the year 2000 [1], compared to 14.2% in 1985. Parallel changes in the population pyramid will necessitate a critical review of the volume and type of services. This is required since in 2000 32% of the population will be either over 64 or below 15 years of age (i.e. dependent population). Thus, for every two persons of the working age population there will be one person in the dependent population [1]. If health insurance premiums are not to grow prohibitively high, compulsory curative types of services may have to be reduced with the aim to concentrate more on high cost, catastrophic care instead of covering all health services, including those for minor ailments. This may also imply that preventive care will have to be focused more and restricted to population groups and conditions for whom it is known to be effective. Thus, due to a more strained financial situation in the health services system, a reduction or redistribution of services may be required.

The growing proportion of the elderly is expected to trigger further increases in costs of health services, as they currently consume more than their respective population proportion of ambulatory medical care contacts, of hospital days, and of prescribed drugs.

This, however, does not necessarily imply that health care expenditures increases of recent years are explained by increases in the population of the elderly. A recent study for the FRG and for the time period between 1970 and 1980 investigated the increase in health services expenditures and differentiated four factors: inflation, medical reasons, increase of volume of services within the statutory scheme and demographic factors [8]. In this approach the structural change in the population is only one factor among several determinants of health care expenditures. According to that study health services expenditure increases due to demographic factors amounted to 6.7% of nominal expenditure increases between 1970 and 1980 for the FRG [8]. Furthermore, it was found that 17.6% of nominal expenditure increases of the ambulatory medical care sector, 8.7% of expenditure increases of the hospital sector, and 11.3% of the nominal expenditure increases in prescribed drugs were attributable to demographic factors [8]. In that time period the proportion of the elderly in the FRG increased from 13.2% in 1970 to 15.2% in 1981 [1]. Thus, the increase in nominal expenditures due to demographic factors was less than proportional to the increase in the elderly portion of the population.

This implies that demographic factors only partially explain health services expenditure increases. Therefore, demographic and disease monitoring, as G. Wilensky and S. Chapman suggest, may only supply limited information with respect to needs in health services, if other factors, such as general economic development, supply of physicians and other medical personnel, service volume in compulsory schemes, health services financing and physician payment schemes are not monitored at the same time.

Relationship Between the Reduction of Mortality and the Concurrent Trend in Morbidity

As age-specific mortality has been decreasing in the past 100 years, life expectancy has been increasing steadily. However, this process has been slowing down, as the yearly increase in life expectancy was greater around the turn to the 20th century than it is in the 1980s [1]. This relationship may be further quantified by studying the effect of a reduction in mortality on the extension of the lifespan. It may be expressed by a measure suggested by Keyfitz [6]. This indicator (the entropy) was 0.117 for females and 0.151 for males for the FRG [7]. Given this size of entropy, an average decrease in mortality by 10% would result in an average increase of life expectancy at all ages by 10% x 0.117 or 1.17% for females and 1.51% for males. More specifically, a 10% reduction in mortality would have increased the life expectancy of a newborn baby girl by (76.7 x 0.117) about 7.5 months and that of a 75-year-old woman by less than 1 month in 1979/1981 [1]. Analyses have shown that such entropies varied between 0.083 and 0.158 (1 : 1.9) for females, and between 0.108 and 0.202 (factor 1 : 1.9) for males for selected European countries (Sweden, Denmark, France, Czechoslovakia, Federal Republic of Germany, Austria, Spain,

Greece) between 1970 and 1978/79 [7]. The variability of entropies across countries suggests that there may be a substantial variability of entropies within countries as well.

Wilkins and Adams [9] studied the relationship between life expectancy and quality-adjusted (adjusted for disability periods, including their severity) life expectancy. They found that even though an increase in life expectancy could be observed for Canadians between 1951 and 1978, rates of persons with activity restrictions increased during the same time. However, after reducing life expectancy by years in a state of activity limitation, real net gains remained in the time period considered. They were 3 years of additional quality-adjusted years of life for Canadian males and 6 years for Canadian women in the time period between 1951 and 1978 [9]. In that same period life expectancy of newborns increased by 4.5 years for males and by 7.5 years for females. Thus, while life expectancy of newborns was increased by 6% for males and by 10.6% for females, quality-adjusted life expectancy increased by 4.2% for males and by 8.2% for females in Canada between 1951 and 1978. While there seems to be a trade-off between decreases in mortality and increasing functional limitations, it is only a partial one, and these net gains in quality-adjusted life expectancy differed by sex, income and size of city. Thus, as G. Wilensky and S. Chapman suggest, the relationships between life expectancy and disability-free life expectancy are complex, as they are influenced by a multitude of variables.

Distribution of Health Services Use Within Countries

Recent cross-sectional and longitudinal studies have shown differences in mortality rates within a population by income for the USA [4] and by socio-economic variables for England, such as ownership of a house or car [2]. Hadley [3] found that greater medical care use contributes significantly to lower mortality rates. He estimated that a 10% increase in per capita medical care use decreases mortality by about 1.5%. He derived these results from the analysis of cohort data.

If income, other socio-economic variables and level of health services use are positively or even causally related to mortality rates, then health services systems have to examine the level and the range of these variables within the health services component of their countries. If the level of these variables is lower than in countries of similar degrees of industrialization, then policy might be directed at reducing barriers to access to health services use. If differences are high between low and high regions or different population groups within the same country by socio-economic variables, rates of use, and mortality, then, for reasons of equity, strategies for removing the gaps in use rates should be developed. If Hadley's findings can be generalized, then strategies for narrowing the range between low and high health services use rates should be devised. If this were achieved by elevating low use rates, then the general level of the health services use rate would be increased and this would presumably reduce mortality in the future. Thus, such inequities within and across countries measure an aspect of need which may not be described by demographic and disease monitoring alone. It needs to be supplemented by information documenting the reasons for the differences. Knowing that the general level of use in the industrialized countries is relatively high already, focussing on the variablity of use and its determinants may be very important. Explanatory factors for these differences are to be found on the demand and on the supply side. According to Kamper-Jorgensen [5], the demand side has been carefully analyzed and barriers to access were substantially reduced. He suggests more focus now on the supply side. According to him, determinants of health services supply differences are not yet sufficiently understood and it will be difficult to do any relevant monitoring in this respect.

Summary

Comments on G. Wilensky's and S. Chapman's paper "Demographic indicator systems of health care needs" were presented in relation to three aspects:

1. While the importance of changing population structure by age and sex as determinants of health services expenditures in years to come cannot be denied, the influence of other factors, such as economic situation, values, organization of health services, financing of services and payment of physicians may be equally important or even more so as determinants of the increase of health services expenditures.

2. As decreasing mortality has been changing the population structure by age and sex, disability and disease patterns in the population will most probably be modified. We still need to better understand the relationship between these phenomena and how they affect different population subgroups and different age cohorts. Thus, I agree with G. Wilensky and S. Chapman on the fact that monitoring precursors of disease, morbidity, disability and mortality in a coordinated fashion might yield information about changing health services needs which is not currently available in sufficient quality, quantity and detail.

3. Empirical studies show that there still exists substantial variability in mortality and morbidity within industrialized countries. Such variability may be partially explained by prior variability in health services use. As the demand determinants of use are reasonably well-known, the supply determinants should now get more attention. In this state of development, focused monitoring is not possible, as the relationships between supply and use of health services are not sufficiently known in detail.

References

1. Der Bundesminister für Jugend, Familie und Gesundheit: Daten des Gesundheitswesens. Ausgabe 1983. Schriftenreihe des Bundesministers für Jugend, Familie und Gesundheit, Band 152. Kohlhammer, Stuttgart 1983

2. Fox, A.J. and Goldblatt, P.O.: 1971-1975 Longitudinal Study of Socio-demographic Mortality Differentials. Series LS, No. 1. Office of Population Censuses and Surveys. Her Majesty's Stationary Office, London 1982

3. Hadley, J.: More Medical Care, Better Health? The Urban Institute, Washington, D.C., 1982

4. Hadley, J. and Osei, A.: Does Income Affect Mortality? Medical Care 20 (9), 1982

5. Kamper-Jorgensen, F.: Causes of Differences in Utilization of Health Services in the Scandinavian Countries. Scandinavian Journal of Social Medicine. Supplement 32, 1984

6. Keyfitz, N.: Applied Mathematical Demography. Wiley, New York 1977

7. Schach, E.: Health Status of the Population: Changes in the Past and Predictions for the Future. Paper prepared for the International Conference on the Future of Health and Health Systems in Industrialized Societies, May 1985

8. Schwartz, F.-W., Robra, B.-P., Heuser, M.R., Henke, K.-D. und Behrens, C.S.: Medizinische Orientierungsdaten. Zentralinstitut für die Kassenärztliche Versorgung, Köln 1983

9. Wilkins, R. and Adams, O.: Healthfulness of Life. The Institute for Research on Public Policy, Montreal 1983

7. Some Remarks on the Applied Theory of Heterogeneous Populations

Alexander Petrovski

The development of noncommunicable diseases in aging populations is highly influenced by risk factors. Individuals react differently to the risk factors and therefore the population (cohort) becomes non-homogeneous. Several long-term indicators might be considered as functionals of risk factors. An example is the known fact that the number and distribution in time of child births determine the probability for a woman to get breast cancer at a given age.

The theory of heterogeneous populations, which is now under development in the International Institute for Applied Systems Analysis, Laxenburg, Austria (IISA) and scientific groups in the USSR and USA, is a suitable analytic tool to handle the problem of resource allocation in screening for noncommunicable diseases among the subgroups of individuals in the whole population.

Based on the above-mentioned functionals as long-term indicators of the health status of individuals, a strategy of screening may be constructed. This strategy will realize a much higher sensitivity of screening than any strategy based on the assumption that the population is homogeneous.

Some papers presented at the session on "Policy Analysis for Cancer Control" during the Third International Conference on System Science in Health Care show us that at present we are near to the threshold effect: a little improvement in screening sensitivity will be followed by a considerable economic effect [1].

The theory of heterogeneous populations itself was presented by A.I. Yashin and me at the sessions on "Health System Modelling" and on "Health System Performance Indicators" during the above-mentioned conference [2; 3].

References

1. Eimeren van, W., Engelbrecht, R. and Flagle, Ch. D. (eds): Third International Conference on System Science in Health Care. Springer-Verlag, Berlin Heidelberg New York Tokyo 1984

2. Petrovski, A. M.: Mathematical Modelling of the Dynamics of Health Indicatos. In: Eimeren van, W., Engelbrecht, R. and Flagle, Ch. D. (eds): System Science in Health Care. Springer-Verlag, Berlin Heidelberg New York Tokyo 1984, pp. 1058-62

3. Petrovski, A. M., Vaupel, J. W., Yashin, A. I.: Models of Risk Group Dynamics. In: Eimeren van, W., Engelbrecht, R. and Flagle, Ch. D. (eds): System Science in Health Care. Springer-Verlag, Berlin Heidelberg New York Tokyo 1984, pp. 936-7

8. Projecting Long-Term Trends in Health Manpower: Methodological Problems

Uwe E. Reinhardt

Health care is one of those basic commodities whose adequate provision is taken to be the responsibility of government. This does not mean that a nation's health care facilities must necessarily be owned by government or that health professionals need be government employees. It merely implies that government bears the ultimate responsibility for an adequate supply of health services, whatever privately or publicly owned instruments it may rely upon in fulfilling that responsibility.

Given this responsibility, it is only natural that public policy-makers seek information on the future demand for and supply of health manpower of various types, particularly of physicians. Usually the forecasts being sought are set within horizons of 10 to 20 years – enough time, it is thought, to allow remedial action should future imbalances be detected. In the United States, attempts to provide such forecasts go back to the early 1930s when Lee and Jones [5] assessed future physician requirements on the basis of detailed epidemiological analyses, a truly pioneering effort for that time. In the meantime, the publication of health manpower forecasts has occurred with regularity.

The track record of these efforts has been mixed. In a critical review of American health manpower forecasts published during the 1950s and 1960s, Lee Hansen [4] showed that forecasters had consistently underestimated both the future demand for and the future supply of physicians. Although I am not familiar with health manpower forecasting in other nations, it is a safe bet that rather large forecasting errors have occurred there as well. One can think of several reasons for such errors.

First, to cite an old adage of unknown origin, "everthing is hard to predict, especially the future". As will be illustrated further on in this essay, the time path of the demand for and the supply of health services is shaped by a myriad of factors whose precise separate and joint influence is not known and, just as importantly, whose future time path also remains a matter of conjecture. Policy-makers in the field often expect too much from health manpower forecasters, and the latter occasionally (and immodestly) promise too much. The best any health manpower forecast can ever achieve, even under ideal circumstances, is a rough indication of major future trends that might occur in the absence of policy intervention, and rough indications of what might occur under alternative scenarios – e.g., in response to alternative policy interventions.

Second, a reason why the predictions of health manpower forecasters are frequently off the mark lies precisely in their usefulness: they tend to trigger remedial policy interventions designed to redress whatever future imbalances have been detected. For example, one reason why earlier forecasters in the United States have so often underestimated the future supply of physicians probably reflects the fact that supply was augmented in response to a predicted manpower shortage.

Third, policy-makers frequently demand and forecasters supply *normative* projections indicating the demand for health services that would be manifest if the need for medical intervention were always correctly perceived by individual patients and translated by them into effective demand, that is demand backed up by a willingness to seek and to accept appropriate health services and an ability to pay for them. This ideal translation from objective need to effective demand is not invariably made. For that reason alone, any normative health manpower forecast may be far off the demand and supply pattern that will actually obtain.

In the remainder of this essay, these problems will be explored in greater depth, with emphasis on certain conceptual and methodological aspects of health manpower forecasting. The objective of the paper is to alert the users of such forecasts to the complexity of the enterprise, and to its inherent limitations, lest more be expected from the research community than can reasonably be delivered.

Basic Analytic Steps and Concepts in Health Manpower Forecasting

The basic analytic steps in any manpower forecast are always the same. One begins with a projection of the nation's future population, broken down as finely as is possible into socio-demographic groups. Given this projection one must, next,

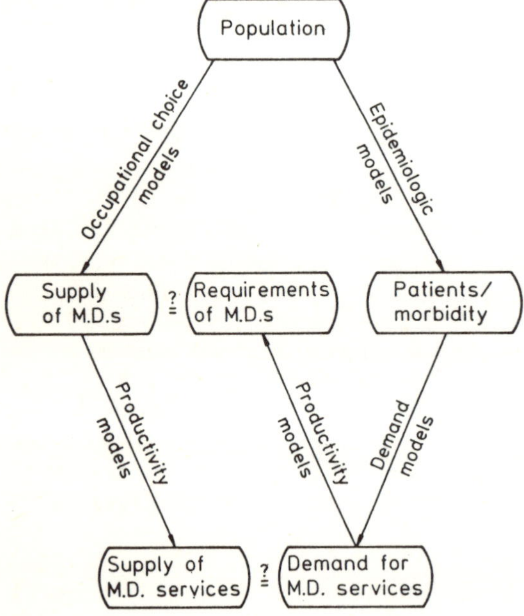

Fig. 1. Schematic overview of health manpower forecasting

translate it into (a) the supply of health manpower most likely to be yielded by the projected population and (b) the demand for health services most likely to be generated by that same population. Figure 1 illustrates this process in the most rudimentary way for medical doctors. In Fig. 2, that process is restated in the form of a basic forecasting equation that highlights the several variables whose future values must be projected by health manpower forecasters to detect potential future imbalances. That equation alone should persuade the reader of the enormous complexity of even the simplest health manpower forecast.

The ultimate objective of any health manpower forecast is, of course, to gain a perspective on the future balance between the demand for and supply of *health services*. As Fig. 1 makes clear, one may explore that issue by translating projected population figures into the associated morbidity, and then translating the expected morbidity into a corresponding need or demand for health services. By means of a production model, the demand for health services is then translated into the implied *required number of physicians*. Finally, the required number of physicians is contrasted with the projected supply of medical manpower to identify potential future imbalances. In Fig. 2, the projected imbalance (if any) is denoted by variable X_t.

In what follows, it will be useful for illustrative purposes to continue the discussion of health manpower forecasting primarily with reference to *physician manpower*. Further on, we can relax that restriction to consider also the interdependence

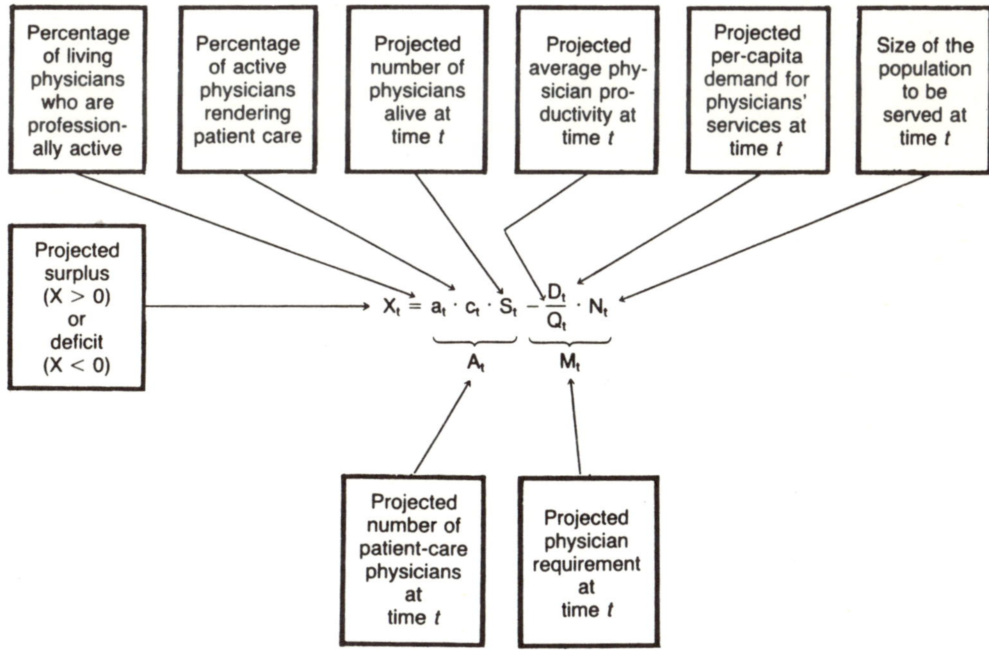

Fig. 2. A simple forecasting equation for physician manpower

among different types of manpower, for example, the effect of physician support staff on physician productivity.

Projecting the Future Supply of Physician Services

In a democratic society that affords its people freedom of occupational choice, the future supply of any given type of manpower likely to emerge from future cohorts of young individuals can be predicted only with the aid of empirically estimated models of occupational choice. The current state of the art of such models leaves them rather imprecise, for obvious reasons.

First, at any point in time, the occupational choices of young individuals are likely to be influenced by a whole host of factors, only some of which are quantifiable and predictable. In their models, economists have tended to stress economic variables, such as the expected future income from a profession and the cost of entering it. While these variables have been shown to be influential at the margin, they furnish only partial explanations of occupational choice. Prevailing social ethics, the prestige of a profession and mere fads are easily as important.

Occupational choice models can, at best, predict the future demand for professional training. To predict the actual supply of trained manpower requires forecasts also of the supply of professional training and of the interaction between demand and supply. In most of the European nations, the supply of professional training is determined by ministries of education, often in abstraction from future manpower requirements. The supply thus emerges from an essentially political decision. By contrast, in the United States public funds underwrite only part of the cost of professional training. While the public sector can influence the overall capacity of professional schools, it cannot fully determine that capacity. At this time, for example, an increasing number of Americans purchase medical education abroad – in Europe, Israel, Mexico or the for-profit Caribbean medical schools.

Finally, even if one could predict the future time path of medical graduates likely to emerge from a nation's medical-school system, there remains one further important source of medical manpower: immigration. In the United States, that sourcehas furnished a very substantial number of medical graduates: close to 50% of all new physicians in some years during the 1970s. In Europe that source has been important as well. Of particular concern to the manpower planners of any given nation must be the freedom physicians of the European community have to move across national frontiers.

In short, then, while it may seem easy at first blush to predict the future supply of physicians 10 or 20 years hence, in practice such forecasts are fraught with uncertainty, especially if the projections are disaggregated into distinct medical specialties. Past forecasts have tended to be rather wide of the mark in this area. Having learned from the experience, modern practitioners of forecasting usually furnish an entire range of forecasts – certainly a high, medium and low forecast. Policymakers in the field may find this ambiguity unsettling. It is, however, the best any careful forecaster could possibly do.

Once the supply of physicians has been projected for future years, that supply must be translated into the corresponding number of *physicians services*. This requires one, first, to define an operationally meaningful measure of output and, second, to develop a production model capable of converting numbers of physicians into number of physician hours worked and thence into the number of physician services produced per physician per period of time (e.g. year).

One of the major difficulties encountered in health manpower forecasting is that the definition of the physician's output is so elusive. A physician's practice is really a multi-product firm that produces an entire vector of distinct services. In principle, the projected morbidity pattern must be translated into the corresponding set of health services required or demanded at future points in time, and the quantity of each distinct type of service must then be translated into the corresponding demand for health manpower. Such ambitious forecasts have on occasion been attempted, most recently, in the United States, by the US Graduate Medical Education National Advisory Committee (GMENAC), an advisory body to the Secretary of the US Department of Health and Human Services (see [3]). Such detailed forecasts, however, require substantial input of financial and human resources. A shortcut, which may be quite acceptable in practice, has been to base the forecast on the predominant element of the health services vector, on the assumption that other elements of the vector are closely and positively related with that dominant element. In the case of physicians, for example, many forecasters have based their projections simply on estimated future office visits by patients, perhaps broken down by physician specialty. Given the observed secular stability in the per-capita utilization of office visits by particular socio-demographic groups, the assumption is that office visits are a reasonably good index for the physician's overall output of services (for a lengthier justification of this shortcut, see [11]). Figure 2 implicitly adopts that shortcut.

In Fig. 2, the translation of the projected future supply of physicians into the probable number of office visits to be had from that supply is represented by the productivity variable Q_t, thought of there as the annual number of office visits that can be handled, on average, per physician at some future time t. This productivity variable is a crucial determinant of the future supply of medical services. It therefore behooves health manpower forecasters to research the determinants of that productivity variable with the utmost care.

The average number of medical services a physician can produce in a given period depends, in the first instance, upon the support staff assisting him or her. Just what effect support staff has on, say, the number of patients physicians can see per hour can be estimated with empirical production functions which relate the physicians visit-rate mathematically to the number of hours worked by the physician, the number of hours of time spent by support staff and yet other inputs – for example, the number of examination rooms at the physician's disposal. Table 1, taken from Reinhardt [11] illustrates the potential trade-off between physician time and that of support staff for the American context. That table is based on production-function estimates extracted from a large nation-wide sample of office-based physicians (see [10]). The data in the table indicate that, up to a point, the delegation of tasks from the physicians to support staff can increase the physician's own pro-

Table 1. Estimated technically feasible trade-offs between office-based physicians and support personnel in the United States, 1970 and 1990[a]

		Number of physicians and support personnel required if the number of aides per physician (L) is equal to					
		0	1	1.75	2.0	3.0	4.0
Estimated annual rate of office visits		2850	3391	4821	5124	6311	7345
per physician[b] (Index set equal to 1.00 for $L = 1.75$)		0.59	0.82	1.00	1.06	1.31	1.5
1970							
Size of resident population:	204 million						
Average annual visits per capita:	4.6[c]						
No. of MDs required ('000s)		326	236	192	181	147	126
No. of aides required ('000s)		0	236	337	362	441	505
1990							
Size of resident population:	245 million[d]						
(a) Zero growth in per capita demand:							
Average annual visits per capita:	4.6						
No. of MDs required ('000s)		391	283	231	217	176	152
No. of aides required ('000s)		0	283	404	434	529	606
(b) Annual growth in per capitademand:	3%						
Average annual visits per capita:	8.3						
No. of MDs required ('000s)		712	516	421	396	321	276
No. of aides required ('000s)		0	516	736	792	964	1104

[a] Based on the assumption that physicians in 1970 employed the equivalent of the time of 1.75 aides each
[b] Based on the productivity index for the office-visit equation estimated from the sample of internists
[c] Office visits only
[d] Office-based MDs rendering patient care

Source: Reinhardt [11], Table 7-4, p. 204

ductivity quite substantially. Just how far that process can be pushed in a particular country or region depends, of course, on the prevailing practice pattern. In the United States, that potential appears to have been all but exploited when support staff reaches a size of between five and six persons per physician. Because support staff is expensive, however, the *economic* potential to exploit task delegation (as distinct from its strictly *technical* feasibility) is already fully exploited between three and four support staff per physician.

Whatever the case may be in a particular country, however, it is surely the case that there does not exist a hard-and-fast optimal ratio of physicians needed to serve any given population adequately. To make that point is the main objective of Table 1. We shall return to it further on, in the Section "Potential Trade-Offs in the Production of Health Care".

Quite aside from the effect support staff has on the productivity of physicians, their gender appears to have a pronounced influence on their hourly patient load as well. Tables 2 to 4 illustrate this phenomenon for the United States. These tables are based, once again, on a large, nation-wide cross section of office-based physicians surveyed in 1981. It is seen that, on average, female physicians see only 75% as many patients per year than do their male counterparts. Figures 3 and 4 illustrate the same phenomenon for France, where the differential appears to be even wider (see [2]). In an earlier study of general practictioners in the Canadian province of Quebec, that differential was detected as well. After controlling for all other practice inputs (including support staff), it was found that female physicians tended to see an average of about 30% fewer patients per hour than did their male colleagues (see [1]).

The reasons for these gender-related productivity differentials have not been well explored so far, perhaps because the subject matter is rather delicate (certainly in the United States). It is possible that the phenomenon is transitory – that the differential will disappear once a larger number of women have entered into the med-

Table 2. Average number of office visits per year by gender of physician: general practitioners in the United States in 1981

Variable	Male (n=587)	Female (n=39)	Female Male
Office visits/hour	3.78	2.78	0.73
Hours per week devoted to office visits	33.26	32.76	0.97
No. of weeks in practice/year (1981)	47.39	44.25	0.93
Estimated office visits/year[a]	5958	4030	0.68

[a] Calculated as office visits/hour x office hours/week x weeks/year

Source: Data provided by the American Medical Association

Table 3. Average number of office visits per year by gender of physician: specialists in internal medicine in the United States in 1981

Variable	Male (n=549)	Female (n=46)	Female Male
Office visits/hour	2.45	1.99	0.81
Hours per week devoted to office visits	27.18	25.19	0.92
No. of weeks in practice/year (1981)	46.43	43.15	0.92
Estimated office visits/yeara	3092	2163	0.70

[a] Calculated as office visits/hour x office hours/week x weeks/year

Source: Data provided by the American Medical Association

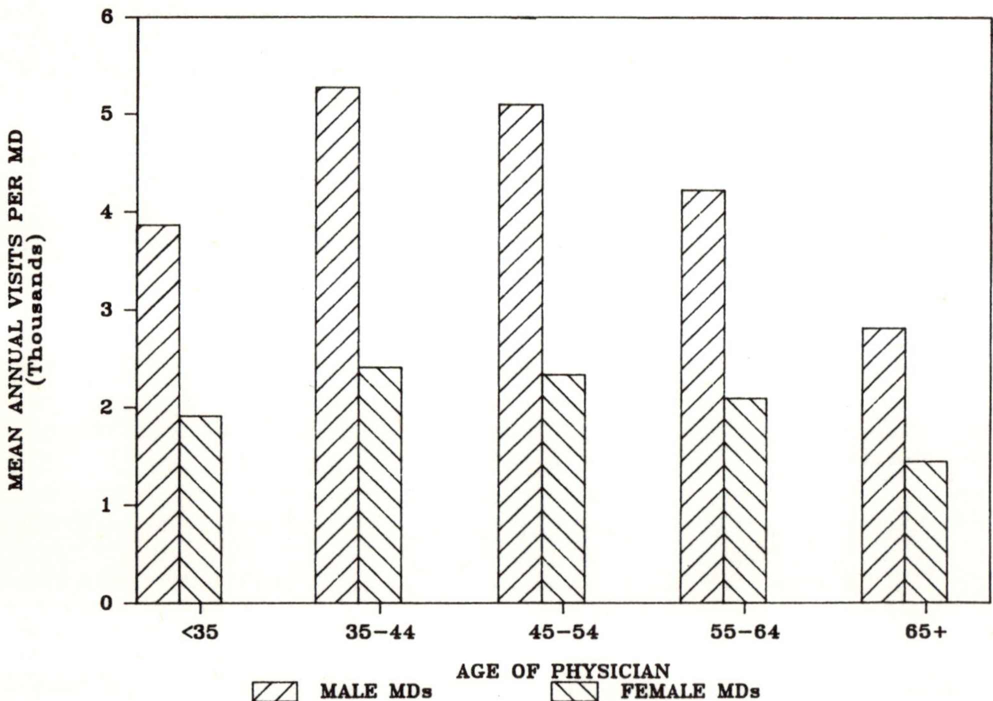

Fig. 3. Patient load of French physicians in 1981by age and sex of physicians (from [2], Table 46, p.93)

Table 4. Average number of office visits per year by gender of physician: pediatricians in the United States in 1981

Variable	Male (n=204)	Female (n=59)	Female Male
Office visits/hour	3.19	3.08	0.97
Hours per week devoted to office visits	33.67	27.44	0.81
No. of weeks in practice/year (1981)	47.22	45.27	0.95
Estimated office visits/yeara	5072	3826	0.75

[a] Calculated as office visits/hour x office hours/week x weeks/year

Source: Data provided by the American Medical Association

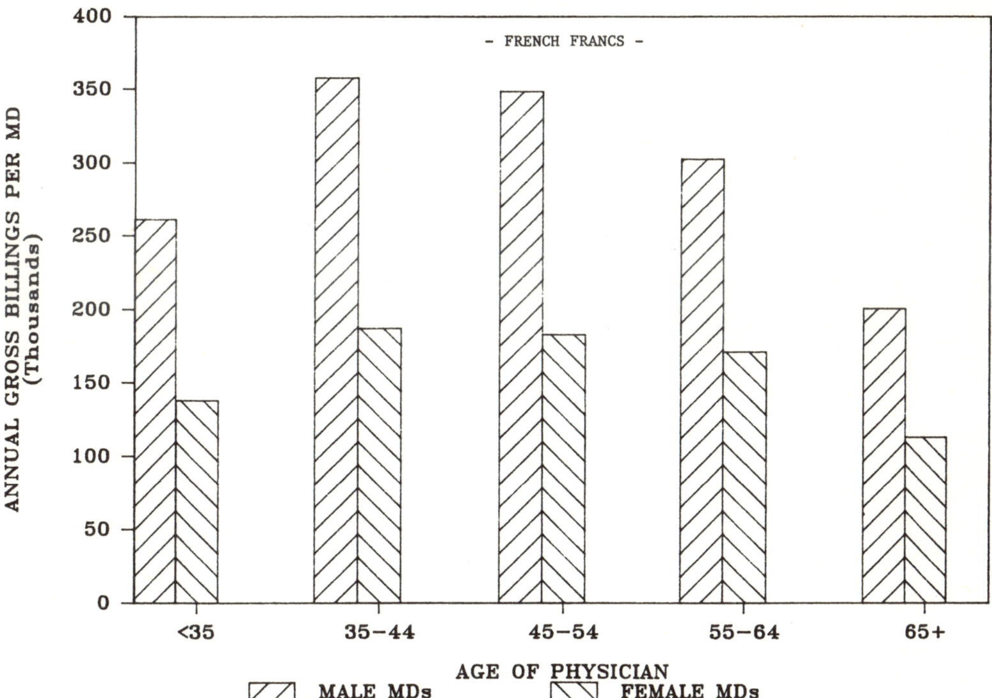

Fig. 4. Gross billings of French MDs in 1981 by age and sex of physicians (from [2], Table 46, p.93)

ical profession. In the meantime, however, manpower forecasters would be remiss in their task were they to abstract from this phenomenon in their projections. At this time, it is still reasonable to assume that a projected physician supply that includes a relatively high proportion of female physicians will represent a smaller supply of medical services than will a similar-sized number of predominantly male physicians.

Figures 3 and 4 illustrate one further factor affecting physician productivity in any country: the average age of the physician stock. Both the hourly rate of patient visits and the number of hours physicians work per year appears to trace out an inverted U-shaped curve reaching a maximum somewhere between age 45 and 50 (although the peak may well vary from country to country). In translating a given number of physicians into the corresponding supply of medical services, attention should therefore be paid to the age composition of the physician stock as well.

Finally, in making long-run projections of health manpower, researchers must forever be mindful that the clinical content of medical treatments changes over time in a manner that may alter the relationship between required health services and required health manpower. That point, however, is more fruitfully discussed in connection with the demand for health services to which we shall now turn.

Projecting Future Physician Requirements

The crudest approach to projecting future physician requirements is simply to multiply projected future population by some target physician-population ratio. The target ratio may be either the prevailing national average, or some normative ratio – for example, the ratio prevailing in the most generously endowed regions of the nation. Because it is easily understood by laypersons, and also because it is inexpensive, that approach has been widely used in health manpower forecasting. But the approach has obvious shortcomings. It projects a static picture of morbidity and of medical technology.

Ideally, as noted earlier, one would like to project the future morbidity pattern likely to be generated by projected future populations, translate this morbidity pattern into required health services and, finally, into the implied health manpower requirements. That more sophisticated approach, for example, was adopted by Lee and Jones [5] and, more recently, by the previously cited (GMENAC). That committee's final report, published in 1980, represents the latest large-scale health manpower forecast published in the United States [3] . Because that forecast certainly ranks as the most ambitious such project ever to come forth in the United States, it may merit a brief synopsis at this point. (A more extended description of the project can be found in [9] .)

The first step in the GMENAC model was the projection of the total burden of disease and disability of the United States population for the target year of 1990. These projections were based on a great variety of local, national and international epidemiological data bases. With the aid of Delphi panels drawn from the relevant medical specialties, the projected future morbidity (expressed as X number of cases of a particular condition per year) was then translated into "true need" for medical interventions. This translation was based on what was considered by the Delphi panels as "good standards of care", but not "utopian standards". Included in the projection of "true need" were preventive services thought to be efficacious.

In terms of our forecasting equation in Fig. 2, this exercise thus yielded normative projections for the total number of required health services, $D_t \, . \, N_t$, broken down by type of medical service. For ambulatory services, the unit of service needed was defined as encounters between patients and physicians or their staffs. For inpatient services, the units of service were either operations and/or inpatient days.

Having projected the total set of specific medical interventions assumed by the Delphi panels to be "needed" by the United States population in 1990, the GMENAC forecasters next translated these services requirements into the implied manpower requirements. This translation was not based on currently prevailing practice patterns, but on models of efficient task assignments among different types of health manpower (physicians, physician support staff, physical therapists, and so on). In terms of Fig. 2, this translation reflects itself in a normative value of Q_t for each type of medical manpower.

By dividing the projected service requirements ($D_t \, . \, N_t$) by the corresponding productivity index (Q_t) for each medical specialty, the GMENAC then arrived at the number of medical specialists of each type "needed" by 1990. That "need" was then contrasted with the projected supply to detect potential future imbalances in supply and demand.

In principle, the approach used by the GMENAC has considerable appeal. In its application, however, the approach is only as reliable as are the Delphi panels implementing it. The respect with which such a forecast is greeted depends crucially on the stature of the Delphi panels. These problems notwithstanding, resort to Delphi panels may easily yield forecasts as valid as any other based on more scientifically rigorous estimation methods, particularly when the latter are applied on historical data that may reflect an obsolete structural context.

Potential Pitfalls in Health Manpower Forecasting

Two major shortcomings have plagued health manpower forecasts in the past. The first of these has been excessive reliance on *normative* rather than *positive* models. The second has been excessive reliance on *point estimates* without adequate sensitivity analysis.

Normative vs Positive Forecasting

Early in the development of a health manpower forecast researchers must decide whether their forecasts are to be their best, educated guess of actual future developments or the manpower picture that would obtain under ideal circumstances.

Forecasts based upon epidemiological data tend to be of the latter variety. As was illustrated above with reference to the GMENAC forecast, it is possible to translate projected morbidity into "true, objective need" for medical interventions, with the necessary "objectivity" being furnished by panels of medical experts. In spite of their appeal, however, such models remain essentially organized efforts at wishful thinking. Ultimately, the experts' normative assessments of the "need" for medical intervention is irrelevant if patients themselves are unwilling or unable to translate the *need* for intervention into what economists call *effective demand*, that is, actual demand for medical intervention backed up by both a willingness and an ability to pay for such interventions. For that reason a realistic forecast of the future health manpower picture can emerge only from an amalgam of *epidemiological* and *economic* models of the demand for health services. In terms of the forecasting equation in Fig. 2, this means that the projected per-capita demand D_t should emerge from an economist's empirical demand function (which will, of course, include socio-demographic and epidemiological variables) and not simply from the expert judgement of epidemiologists and physicians (unless, of course, policy-makers are genuinely interested in the number of physicians that would have to be made available to satisfy these experts).

Among the economic variables influencing the translation of morbidity into the effective demand for medical interventions are the following:

1. The money price patients must pay for health services at the point of using such services
2. The time price patients must bear to use health services
3. The amenities accompanying the delivery of health services
4. The relative scarcity or abundance of the supply of medical manpower
5. The manner in which physicians and hospitals are paid for rendering health services

In many of the European nations and in Canada, national health insurance systems have effectively reduced to zero the money price patients pay for health services. However, in other countries – for example, France, the United States and Australia – patients still pay a sizeable proportion of the health bill out of pocket at time of service. Extensive research in the United States, spanning a decade or more, has shown rather conclusively that, other things being equal, the effective demand for health services, including hospital admissions, is highly sensitive to the money price borne by patients. In short, projections of the future demand for health services must be based either explicitly or implicitly upon a projected time path of the money prices for health care borne directly by patients in future years.

The relative scarcity or abundance of health-care resources (manpower and facilities) influences the time price patients must bear to access health services, and also the amenities accompanying that care. As the physician-population ratio rises throughout the industrialized world, for example, one must expect physicians to be more attentive to their patients' desire to procure health services with a minimum waste of time and with dignity and comfort. Aside from explicit advertising (which is permitted in the United States) physicians will "advertise" their services through these variables, which are perceived by patients as part of the quality of care. Other things being equal, a reduction in the time price of health care and an increase in amenities must be expected to increase the demand for health services.

Quite aside from the influence of time price and amenities on patients' demand for health services, a relative abundance of physicians and of hospital beds can increase the demand for health services also through a mechanism known as "supplier-induced demand", that is, demand artificially created by health-care providers in order to generate revenue. Just how much latitude physicians and hospitals have to induce demand in this way has long been a matter of controversy, certainly among American health economists. (For a review of the pertinent literature in the United States, see Reinhardt [12] .) Whatever the significance of the effect may be, however, anyone interested in projecting the actual future demand for health services must incorporate some assumption about that significance in his or her forecast.

Closely related to the preceding point is the fifth factor listed above, namely, the manner in which physicians and hospitals are compensated for their services. In their public posturing, physicians and hospital administrators tend to pretend that, in their decisions concerning a patient's treatment, they are motivated strictly by medical criteria and never by financial incentives. It can be doubted that, in the privacy of their own circles, either of them actually believe their own rhetoric on this point. As current experiments with hospital reimbursement in the United States amply demonstrate, hospitals are highly sensitive indeed to the manner in which they are paid. If they receive their revenues in the form of fixed per-diem charges (or in the form of retrospective full-cost reimbursement), then they tend to prolong length of stay per episode of illness. On the other hand, if hospitals are paid a flat fee per diagnostically defined case (as is now the case in the United States), then length of stay for given types of cases can be observed to decline drastically, as it has in the United States. One can expect a similar reaction among physicians. Their treatment decisions are apt to be highly sensitive as well to the marginal profit inherent in additional tests or procedures. (For an overview of this issue, see Reinhardt [13] .)

Normative forecasts of the future need for health services tend to abstract from these and other variables whose time path will shape the actual future demand for health services. If one is interested in *predictions* of future demand, then a normative approach to modeling can easily be misleading.

Normative criteria can distort not only the projected demand for health services, but also their supply. As already noted, a crucial determinant of that supply for any projected number of physicians is the productivity variable Q_t. In the previously cited GMENAC model, for example, that variable was quantified by expert judgement and based on the assumption of an economically efficient delegation of delegable tasks from physicians to support staff. (That ideal pattern of task delegation may not, in fact, obtain.) Nor can one be sure how many hours per week and per year physicians will work in the future. As was noted earlier, an increasing percentage of female physicians may well reduce the number of hours and physician services yielded by a given future number of physicians. Normative forecasting models may make sense within the so-called command economies in which central planners have the political clout to enforce in the field whatever plan they have developed on the drawing board. In the market economies of the Western democracies, normative manpower models may furnish interesting supplemental information, but they are less useful for the crafting of a health manpower policy. Economists, in any event, generally prefer to develop their forecasts in that context on the basis of projected *effective demand* rather than on the basis of "*true need*" as defined by medical experts, even at the risk of being accused of insensitivity to human need. It is merely a simplification of realism.

The Usefulness of Sensitivity Analysis

Figure 5 offers a diagrammatic version of the forecasting equation in Fig. 2. The coordinates in that diagram are not a Cartesian set of coordinates. Rather, they represent a collage of positive orthants, each of which depicts one major building block in a health manpower forecast. Thus, orthant II represents the projected time path of future population Nt. Orthant III represents the translation of future population into the total demand for health services (the slope of the line in that orthant being the projected per-capita demand for health services). Finally, orthant IV represents the relationship between numbers of physicians and the supply of physician services. The slope of the line in that orthant is the previously discussed productivity parameter Q.

Figure 5 illustrates the sensitivity of the projected physician surplus or shortage to changes in physician productivity. Upon insertion into an electronic computer, the

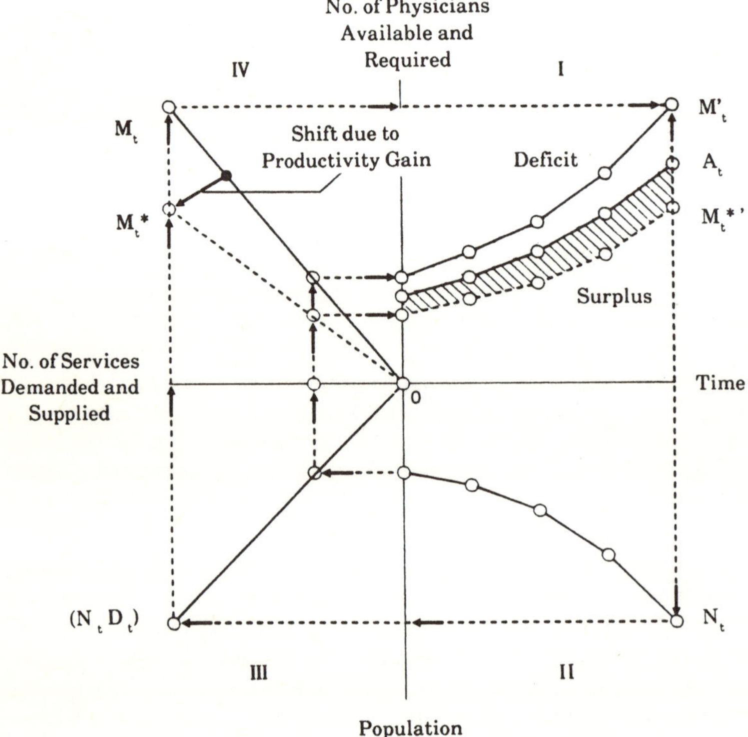

Fig. 5. A rudimentary health manpower forecasting model

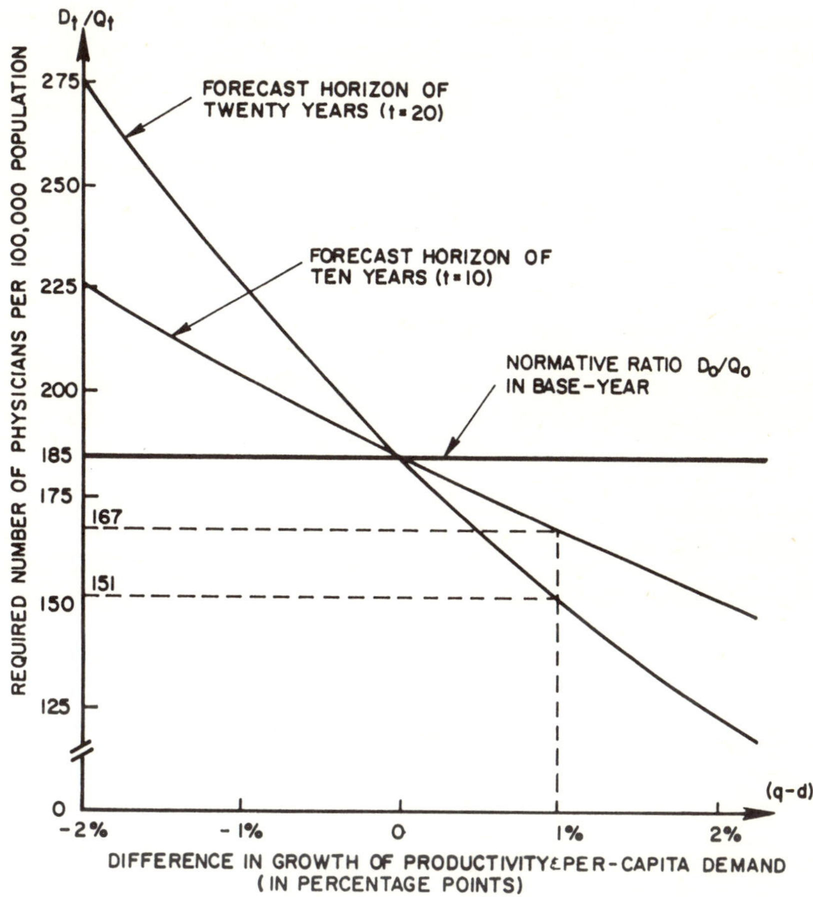

Fig. 6. The sensitivity of future physician requirements to growth in physician productivity

diagram could easily be used to explore the effect of changes in assumptions about yet other variables entering one's manpower forecast explicitly.

Figure 6 illustrates just how sensitive projected health manpower requirements can be to the interplay of assumptions about the future growth in the demand for health services and in the average productivity of physicians. From the forecasting equation in Fig. 2, it emerges that the required future physician-population ratio can be thought of also as the ratio

$$R_t = D_t / Q_t'$$

where D_t denotes the projected future per-capita demand for, say, physician visits and Q_t the number of visits handled per physician per year.

If one denotes by d the projected annual, instantaneous growth rate in the per-capita demand variable D, and by q the corresponding growth rate in the physician productivity variable Q, then the projected future required physician-population ratio can be written as

$$R_t = (D_o / Q_o)e^{-(q-d)t}$$

In Fig. 6, that ratio (R) is plotted on the growth differential ($q - d$) for forecasting horizons of 10 to 20 years. Suppose, for example, one considered the base-year physician-population ratio of 185 physicians per 100 000 population adequate. If the future change in per-capita demand for physician services just equalled the future change in physician productivity, then maintenance of that ratio would be adequate as well. If, on the other hand, the annual growth in per-capita demand outpaced that of physician productivity by 1 percentage point per year, then 226 physicians per 100 000 population would be required 20 years hence, and not only 185. Alternatively, if productivity outpaced per-capita demand by 1 percentage point per year, then only 151 instead of 185 physicians would be required per 100 000 population 20 years hence. Obviously, the longer the forecasting horizon, the more sensitive will be projected physician requirements to changes in the underlying assumptions about d and q.

One could and should undertake similar sensitivity analyses by changing any of the other variables in one's forecasting equation, for example, those listed in Fig. 2. Initially, one might test these one by one. An approach to explore their joint effect might be the following.

For each of the intervening variables shown in the forecasting equation (and perhaps for yet other variables underlying those variables) one might ask appropriate Delphi panels to indicate the lowest and the highest value that could realistically be expected, as well as the most probable value. These suggested values could then be viewed as the parameters of a triangular probability distribution. There would be one distinct such distribution for each variable of interest. Next one would program a computer to draw, say, a million distinct sets of all of the variables in one's forecasting equation, each variable being drawn at random and subject to its own triangular distribution. If there were obvious correlations among sets of variables, these could be built into the simulation. Upon insertion of each of the, say, million distinct sets of variables into the forecasting equation, the target variable X (the projected physician surplus or deficit) would then trace out a frequency distribution that might give one a feel for probable future values of X, given the Delphi panels' expert judgement on the relevant variables. With modern high-speed computers, such simulations would not be difficult, and they could be much refined beyond the mere sketch offered here.

From both the researcher's and the policy-maker's view, simulations of this sort would have a number of virtues.

First, they would convey an idea of the forecast's error of prediction. That error would, of course, not reflect the statistical variance embedded in a body of empirical data, but merely the degree of uncertainty experts assign to a set of projected variables (i.e. the variables entering the forecasting equation). But it would be illuminating, nevertheless.

Second, the simulations can serve to alert the users of health manpower forecasts to the uncertainty necessarily inherent in such exercises, and they can help to protect the forecaster from subsequent criticism. In the sphere of macro-economics, for example, forecasters have opened themselves to much ridicule in recent years by pretending greater accuracy and certainty than fate actually allows the forecaster. Health manpower forecasters would do well to practice their craft with greater caution.

Potential Trade-Offs in the Production of Health Care

In the preceding sections, certain methodological issues arising in health manpower forecasting were illustrated with the aid of a simple forecasting equation strictly for *medical* manpower. As part of that discussion, mention was made of the possibility to substitute one kind of health manpower for another in the production of health services (see Table 1). Actually, possibilities for substitution abound in the health sector. Figure 7, drawn from an earlier paper on the subject [11] illustrates this point.

In Fig. 7, the demand for health services is thought of as the derived demand for one of many inputs into the production of "health status". The health-status production process is managed by the patient, although occasionally with the advice of or even at the command of a physician. As current concerns over "lifestyle" demonstrate, there is increasing appreciating of the trade-offs that exist between medical treatments and other inputs into health-status production. At this time, for example, it is anybody's guess what effect the current emphasis among younger people on health diets and exercise will have on morbidity patterns in the future. To assume that, say, a 77-year-old female in the year 2000 will have, on average, the same demand for health services as does her counterpart today seems highly unrealistic. The link between age-and-sex-specific population groups and the need for health care is anything but tight.

The next set of possible trade-offs occurs at the level of health-care facility. As the experience of the so-called health maintenance organizations and the recent growth of outpatient surgical centers in the United States have shown, there is considerable leeway to substitute ambulatory care for inpatient services in the treatment of given medical cases. This potential trade-off further loosens the link between population and the need for specific health services (e.g. hospital days).

Finally, within each type of health-care facility and in the production of any given type of health service, one type of health manpower can be substituted for another, at least up to a point. That potential trade-off has already been demonstrated earlier with the manpower projections shown in Table 1.

The gist of the preceding comments is that the link between a given population base and the need for a particular type of health manpower required to serve that population adequately is very loose indeed. This conclusion is well illustrated by two sets of empirical observations drawn from the American context.

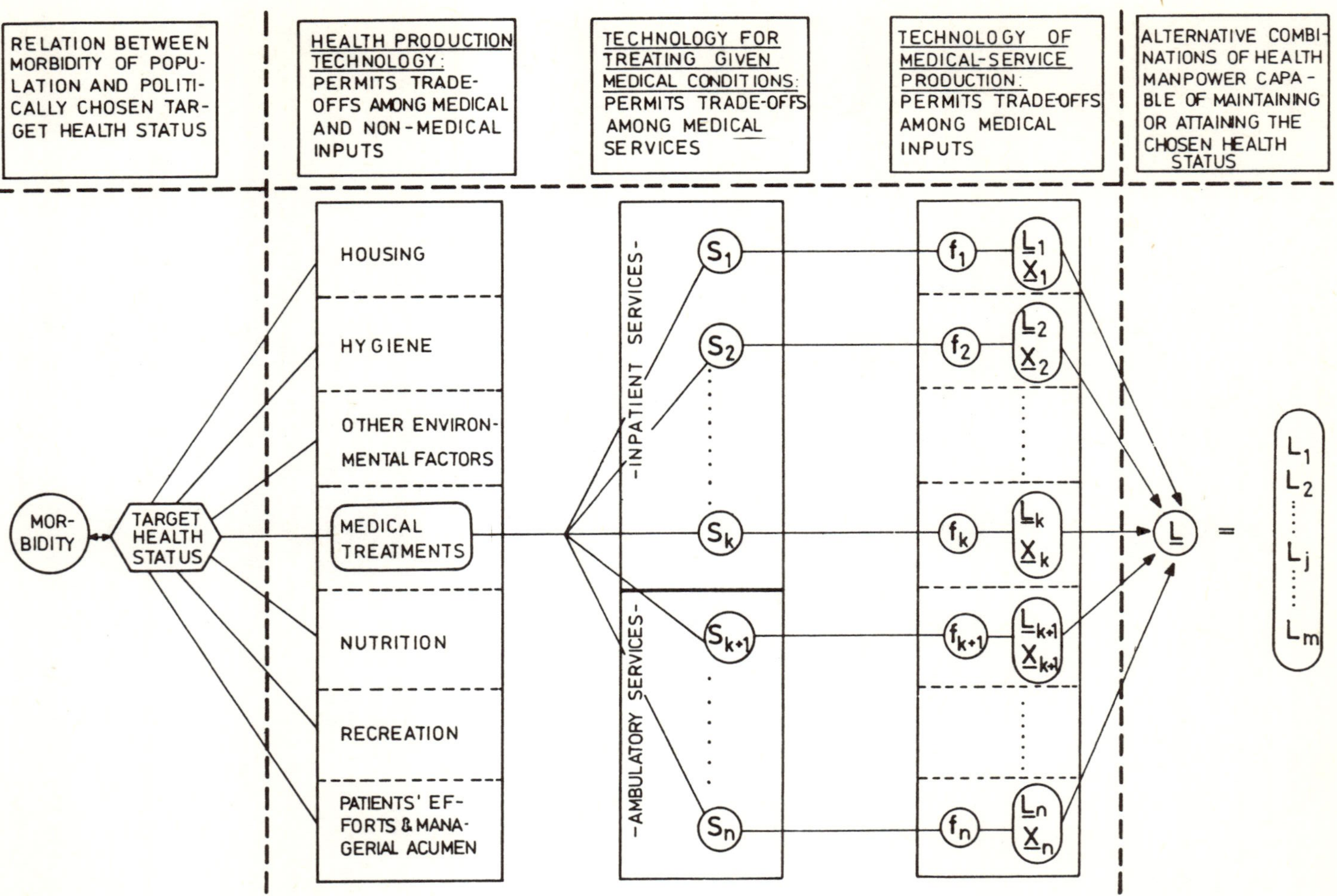

Fig. 7. Potential trade-offs in the production of health

First, as has been found in the pioneering research by John Wennberg et al. [14], there are enormously large and seemingly inexplicable variations across regions in the utilization of health services of seemingly similar populations. Even within as small an area as the New England state of Vermont, the per-capita utilization of services such as hysterectomies, appendectomies and tonsillectomies varies among counties by factors as high as 6 for similar, age-adjusted population groups. So far the only plausible explanation for these extraordinary variations has been that they reflect the preferred "practice style" of physicians. As this essay is written, these variations have attracted the attention of policy-makers at all levels of government, because they imply either that areas with low utilization rates are underserved or, as is more widely believed, that areas with high utilization rates are vastly overserved. In any event, the data show clearly that, for many medical procedures, there is no close link between population groups and the need for particular types of health services. That finding should be disquieting to both health manpower forecasters and to policy-makers in any country.

Second, it has long been known in the United States that health maintenance organizations (which deliver comprehensive health services against prepayment of a flat annual capitation fee) use considerably fewer hospital days per capita to serve their enrolled populations than does the fee-for-service system. Furthermore, while health maintenance organizations typically require one physician per 900 to 1000 enrolled persons, the fee-for-service in the United States system now serves only about 500 patients per physician. These differentials in the use of hospitals and of physician manpower persist even after adjustment for differences in the population being served. Remarkably, no one has yet found any systematic differences in the health status of populations served by health maintenance organizations and by the fee-for-service system (in this connection, see Luft [6] and Manning et al. [8]).

In the literature on health manpower forecasting, one occasionally comes across ambitious enterprises in which the forecaster seeks to project an entire manpower vector M for some future target date t with the aid of a linear model such as

$$M_t = A'D'N_t,$$

where M_t is an mxl vector whose element M denotes the i-type of health manpower required (e.g. hours of time of pediatricians, of physical therapists, of nurses, and so on) at some future target date t, A is an mxn matrix whose element a_{ij} denotes the quantity (e.g. hours) of the i-th type of health manpower (e.g. pediatricians) required to produce one unit of health service type "j ", D is an nxp matrix whose element d_{rs} denotes the average annual per-capita consumption of health service type r by persons in population group s, and N_t is a pxl vector whose element n_s is population group "s ", for example, low-income males aged 50 to 55. (For an example of such a model see Maki [7].) Although such a model appears to be able to forecast simultaneously future requirements for all types of health manpower, it is really nothing other than a stack of separate forecasting equations such as those in Fig. 2, with each equation being completely independent of the other. Furthermore, unless the input-output coefficients a_{ij} are made to vary systematically with time, the model assumes fixed-coefficient production models. In terms of Fig. 2, this implies a constant value over time of the productivity parameter Q_t. Much of this essay has been concerned with the pitfalls of making such an assumption.

To the best of my knowledge, models have not yet been developed that formally incorporate the substitution possibilities sketched out in Fig. 7. To recognize this interdependence formally, one would have to estimate empirically a production function for each distinct type of medical service. In Fig. 7, these functions are denoted by the symbols f_j, $j = 1,...,n$. As already noted, production functions of this type have been estimated for private medical practices, but they do not exist for most other types of health services.

Even if one had the entire set of empirical production functions for all health services, however, jointly these functions would enable one merely to trace out the set of technically feasible, alternative manpower combinations capable of meeting the health-care needs of a population. To conjecture just which combination would actually be attained by the health sector would require one to have an empirically estimated behavioral model of the entire health care sector. No workable, empirical model of this sort exists at this time.

Concluding Observations

Although the preceding caveats may be discouraging, they ought not to daunt the research community. It is a safe bet that policy-makers will continue to request, from time to time, projections of the future health manpower picture. The current state of the art in the field is certainly sufficiently advanced to identify broad trends for, say, 10 to 20 years hence. The models available now also enable policy-makers to explore what-if questions and thus to gain a feel for the impact of alternative policy interventions. While the state of the art in health manpower forecasting is still far from perfect, it shines by comparison with the truly primitive information systems on which our large business firms routinely base their decisions. That fact should be a source of comfort.

References

1. Berry, C.B. et al.: A Study of the Responses of Canadian Physicians to the Introduction of Universal Medical Care Insurance: The First Five Years in Quebec. Mathematica Policy Research, Princeton, NJ, February 1978

2. CREDOC (Centre de Recherche pour l'Etude et l'Observations des Conditions de Vie): Femmes Médicins: Demographie, Activité et Prescriptions en Médicine Liberale. CREDOC, Paris, December 1983

3. GMENAC: Report of the Graduate Medical Education National Advisory Committee to the Secretary of the Department of Health and Human Services. DHHS Publication No. 81-651. Department of Health and Human Services, Hyattsville, Maryland, September 1980

4. Hansen, W.L.: An Appraisal of Physician Manpower Projections. Inquiry 7: 102-113, 1970

5. Lee, R.I. and Jones, L.W.: Fundamentals of Good Medical Care. Chicago University Press, Chicago 1933

6. Luft, H.S.: How Do Health-Maintenance Organizations Achieve Their 'Savings'? New England Journal of Medicine 298: 1336-1343, 25 June 1978

7. Maki, D.R.: A Forecasting Model of Health Manpower Requirements in the Health Occupations. University of Iowa; Industrial Relations Center, Ames, Iowa, 1967

8. Manning, W.G., Leibowitz, A., Goldberg, G.A., Rogers, W.H. and Newhouse, J.P.: A Controlled Trial of the Effect of Prepaid Group Practice on Use of Services. New England Journal of Medicine 310 (23): 1505-1510, June 1984

9. McNutt, D.R.: GMENAC: Its Manpower, Forecasting, Framework. American Journal of Public Health 71: 1116-1124, 1981

10. Reinhardt, U.E.: A Production Function for Physicians Services. Review of Economics and Statistics 54: 55-66, 1972

11. Reinhardt, U.E.: Physician Productivity and the Demand for Health Manpower. Ballinger Publishing Company, Cambridge, Massachusetts, 1975

12. Reinhardt, U.E.: The Theory of Physician-Induced Demand and Its Implication for Public Policy. In: Henke, D. and Reinhardt, U.E.(eds): Steuerung im Gesundheitswesen. Bleicher Verlag, Gerlingen 1983, pp. 150-185

13. Reinhardt, U.E.: Honorierungssysteme in anderen Ländern – Internationaler Vergleich. In: Ferber, C.V., Reinhardt, U.E., Schaefer, H. and Thiemeyer, T. (eds): Kosten und Effizienz im Gesundheitswesen. R. Oldenbourg Verlag, München 1985, pp. 67-94

14. Wennberg, J.E., Barnes, B.A. and Zubkoff, M.: Professional Uncertainty and the Problem of Supplier-Induced Demand. Social Science and Medicine 16: 811-824, 1982

9. Long-Term Trends in Health Care: The Post-Physician Era Reconsidered

Jerrold S. Maxmen

In 1976 I wrote *The Post-Physician Era*[1] in which I predicted that within 50 years, physicians – that is, doctors who diagnose and treat illness – will be rendered obsolete by computers and by allied health personnel, whom I called "medics". I claimed, and still claim, that this development is possible, inevitable and desirable.

This paper summarizes this forecast and some of the reasons behind it. Then, in light of the past 8 years, I re-examine this prediction as it pertains to long-term trends in health care delivery.

Before I start, please understand that I have no specialized expertise in health-care planning, public health or computers. Partly because I am a psychiatrist, what does intrigue me are the social and psychological ramifications of using computers in medicine. Otherwise, computers bore me. I believe that what computers can and should do is frequently overestimated.

The Post-Physician Era: Reviewed

Most papers titled "The Future of *X*" project that if *X* is good and exists, there will be more of *X* in the future. Papers on "The Future of Automobiles" invariably claim we will have more, better and faster cars. Since today's automobiles can go 130 km/h, in the future will they really go 500 km/h? Unlike most predictions, the future is rarely a linear projection of the past. Any thoughtful forecaster considers the emergence of new forces and interactions between new and old forces.

Intelligent forecasting entails more than guessing what may happen. One effective approach is to describe a series of "alternative futures" and to evaluate each by three distinct, yet related, criteria: possibility, inevitability and desirability. An assessment of possibility asks: "*Can* it happen?" An assessment of inevitability asks: "*Will* it happen?" An assessment of desirability asks: "*Should* it happen?" Because something can happen doesn't mean it will happen, and because something will happen, doesn't mean it should happen. These three criteria should always be used to assess any paper on "The Future of *X*".

The Post-Physician Era proposed that over the next 50 years three alternative futures in health-care delivery will evolve. I suggested we will go from the cur-

---

[1] Maxmen JS (1976) *The Post-Physician Era: Medicine in the 21st Century*. Wiley: New York

rently dominant "physician-centered model", in which the doctor makes most of the key medical decisions, to the "health-team model", in which decision-making authority resides with professionals from a variety of health care disciplines, to the "medic-computer model", in which computers (and other high technology) perform the *technical* tasks presently performed by physicians, and allied health personnel called "medics" who perform the *supportive* (e.g. emotional, informational) tasks presently performed by physicians. A post-physician era is possible because eventually every one of the doctors' technical and supportive tasks could be usurped, and if so, what would be left for doctors to do?

Indeed, each of the seven technical tasks of the physicians are *already* being done by technology (sometimes with the help of trained non-physicians), and that even though "medical informatics" is in its infancy, repeated studies demonstrate that computers often conduct these technical tasks better than can physicians. First, computerized *histories* have already been devised which outperform physician-gathered histories. Second, as a valuable source of clinical data, the *physical examination* is rapidly being superseded by far more informative laboratory tests. Third, the ordering and interpretating of *ancillary tests* can already be done by computer. So can the fourth through sixth tasks: *diagnosis, determining treatment, and prognosis*, respectively. The main reason computers are able to conduct these tasks better than physicians is because the ideal performance of these tasks requires three critical features - memory, objectivity, and probability - qualities which machines display far better than humans.

The seventh, and final, technical task is to *implement treatment*, in three general ways: (a) "verbal" interventions, which I argue could be done better by the medics than by physicians; (b) medications – themselves products of technology – which, to update Benjamin Franklin, cure while the doctor takes the fee; and (c) surgery. The last function to be automated – a robot is not about to remove my appendix – is surgery. But given that computer decision-making would greatly reduce the enormous frequency of unneccessary surgery, given that non-physician military corpsmen already perform considerable minor surgery, given that midwives already deliver far more babies than do physicians (in Europe if not yet in America), and given that in the future medications will eliminate the need for many operations (e.g. before 1990 drugs that dissolve gallstones will become available, thereby obviating the need for cholecystectomies) then, gradually, the role of the surgeon will also dissolve.

The medic is crucial to a medic-computer model. His (post-high school) training would be far less costly, taking eighteen months to two years, as opposed to the 12 years required of American physicians. Unlike physicians who are chosen by schools mainly for their scientific abilities, medics would be selected primarily for their interpersonal, psychological, and ethical abilities. (Doctors need to know science and technical facts; medics, armed with the computer, would not.)

Medics would be liaisons between patients and computers: They would discuss the computer's recommendations with the patient, offer information, and address the patient's emotional needs. He or she would also coordinate the patient's medical care, which contrasts sharply with the lack of coordination under the physician-centered and health-team models, in which treatment is split between numerous specialists.

As long as the logical steps which lead to medical decision-making can be delineated, these steps can be, and have been, programed. Unlike physicians who do not always learn from experience, new generations of computers can automatically alter their data bases to provide the most up-to-date services. Under a medic-computer-system, medical researchers would continually revise decision-making programs. Because there will always be legitimate differences over the best way to diagnose and treat patients, just as patients often receive second opinions, in the future, patients could avail themselves of two or more medical decision-making programs.

Unlike now, a medic-computer model could make readily available the very best, most up-to-date, medical expertise to everyone, regardless of geography and income. Since superior medical records would exist, evaluators could better monitor medical care and medics could better serve our increasingly mobile population. Research would improve. At present, virtually all information from the one billion doctor-patient contacts annually gets lost; with a medic-computer model all this information could be saved and used to advance medical knowledge. (To do so, a great many medical researchers will be needed to translate massive amounts of clinical data into clinical software.)

The advent of a post-physician era would radically alter and improve health-care delivery. Regardless of a nation's economic and political systems, as long as physicians are the only ones who have the knowledge to make expert clinical decisions, every health-care system must substantially accommodate to the desires of physicians; with a medic-computer model, the public's needs could have priority.

Although physicians might be expected to resist a medic-computer model, I predict they will hasten it. One reason for this, at least in America, is legal. With the law intruding more and more into the doctor-patient relationship, I keep having this nightmare of a prosecuting attorney drilling me for alleged malpractice: "In treating your patients Dr. Maxmen, are you so arrogant that you don't consult the computerized suggestions from the nation's foremost experts?" If doctors don't want to use automated diagnoses, lawyers will make sure they do.

Beyond this, doctors will also come to depend on computer-generated decisions, feeling it will help provide better care. Patients, who are becoming more familiar with computers, will be asking their doctors to "double-check" with the computer. Some doctors claim that "clinical intuition" gives them a distinct advantage over the machine. Clinical intuition, however, can be wrong as often as right. Doctors are human and make mistakes: sometimes it's because of laziness and carelessness, and sometimes, because their spouse kicked them out of bed the night before. Machines don't have these problems.

Patients will expect their doctor to consult a computer routinely, and with good reason. Charging that medical education is "far too narrow", Derek Bok, the president of Harvard University, pointed to a recent investigation of 100 autopsies "at a prominent teaching hospital", which revealed that doctors made the wrong diagnosis in 22% of the cases, and that "in almost half of such instances, a correct diagnosis might have changed treatment and prolonged life". Another survey of 249 patients in a teaching hospital showed that 20-40% of routine procedures (e.g. examining prostates, analyzing blood sugars, checking stools for blood) were neglected by house staff.

If for no other reason than to feel more confident, patients might want doctors to use computer programs that would prevent neglect by reminding doctors of what to do.[2]

Historically, just as physicians initially felt laboratory tests demeaned their clinical skills only to later embrace and overly depend on them, I predict the same will happen with the computer. The black box will replace the black bag in steps: First, the doctor will use the computer as an aid, then as a routine, and then as a necessity. Eventually, when doctors can no longer practice without it, people will no longer care to practice as physicians. (Because physicians have medical expertise and make critical clinical decisions, whereas medics would not, it would be incorrect to view the medic as simply a "renamed doctor".)

It is silly to have computers do what people can do better, yet equally silly to have people do what computers can do better. A post-physician era allows each to excel at what it does best. Computers are best at making technical decisions. People do best when they offer sick people both comfort and concern, when they encourage patients to adopt healthier habits, and when they help the dying feel less frightened, and their relatives less alone. Only people can bring sensitivity, humanity, wisdom, morality, creativity, and nobility to clincial practice.

The Post-Physician Era: Reconsidered

Since the book's publication, a post-physician era seems far more possible and inevitable, and with less certainty, more desirable. In discussing the book with physicians, I found them amazingly receptive to a medic-computer model. Yet their main reservation surprised me. I had assumed that doctors would like to be freed from the boring, routine tasks of medical practice so they could do tasks that only humans could do. I was wrong: Their greatest worry about computerized medicine was that it would rob them of this routine; doctors were not eager to devote themselves to all that humanism, sensitivity, and ethics, which they keep saying they would love to do "if only I had the time". If they wanted all these wonderful things, they would have gone to philosophy school, not medical school. After I would present them my thesis, doctors would typically say: "With all these computers around I'm going to miss doing the simple things, like taking blood pressures and prescribing drugs." "I like doing what I'm familiar with; I don't want to change." "I'm sure the machines will come, but when they do, what will be left for me to do?" "Your

[2] Reforming the Medical School Curriculum (1984) Update: *Computers in Medicine*, 2(3): 9,19,24,45

medic sounds like a hybrid psychotherapist-ethicist, and that's too ethereal for me. I like medicine because it's concrete and straight-forward."

In my experience, when presented with this forecast, instead of objecting to their obsolescence, physicians have assumed a medic-computer model is possible, inevitable and desirable. They speak of a post-physician era more with resignation than anger. Doctors invariably tell me what they see: Computer terminals popping up in hospital libraries, record rooms, and nurses' stations. In 1976, there was but one journal devoted to computerized medicine – actually a newsletter – today, there are dozens.

Since a post-physician era will not occur overnight, but emerge by lurching more forward than backward, over the next decade the greatest advances in automated medicine will probably be in the creation of software that automatically evaluates health care services in general and clinical outcomes with patients in particular. The only enduring programs will be those which make evaluation an integral component of clinical care, instead of something that is grafted on to it. Since many early efforts at automation failed by not addressing the physician's needs and sensibilities, future programs for evaluation should not get in his way or waste his time; they should give him useful data. For example, if it took relatively little effort, every doctor would love to get a computerized analysis of how his patients are doing in comparison to patients in general with the same demographic, diagnostic and therapeutic variables. With nobody (especially a lawyer) looking over his shoulder, a doctor could find out (for himself) that his diabetics do better than average, but that his epileptics do worse; he could discover his clinical strengths and deficiencies. Already 24-hour-a-day videotext systems are available only for physicians (i.e., Phycom), which provide news of, and answer a doctor's specific questions about, clinical, financial and legal matters pertaining to medicine.

Despite many advances toward a post-physician era *inside* the profession, most have been *outside* of it. For example, back in 1976 there was a serious question of whether laymen might be so afraid of computers they would reject their use in medicine (or in anything). This question is asked no longer.

In retrospect, I greatly underestimated capitalism's ability to induce the public to buy computers, irrespective of whether they need them. (Do I really need a computer to balance my checkbook?) On a typical evening, about one in eight commercials on TV is about computers. Using a word processor is quickly becoming a norm among American college students, for in the modern world, a college student who can't use a computer may well be a functional illiterate. In only the past 5 years, terms like "user-friendly", "floppy disks", and "bits" have taken a byte of our everyday vocabulary. Each month, thousands of people take computer courses to learn about them just "to know what's going on" and "to not feel left out".

Despite the overselling and the overexpectations of the computer, it dominates American life. When *The Post-Physician Era* was published in 1976, I assumed two or more decades would have to pass before people felt sufficiently familiar with the computer to accept a post-physician era; obviously, people's comfort with the machine has arrived much sooner.

As a result, over the next decade there will be an even greater market among the general public for not only health-enhancement programs, but also for automated self-diagnosis and self-treatment. That markets will grow is hardly surprising. As any doctor can tell you, when people call a physician-friend for medical advice, they usually ask: "Should I see a doctor?" or "Is my problem serious?" or "What should I do about it?" When problems are complicated or potentially serious, I tell them to see their doctor. But like most physicians, when friends ask for advice on benign matters, I give it. Yet not everybody personally knows a doctor well enough to get expert advice. With self-help medical software, everybody could get this advice.[3]

Abetted by the flood of home health kits[4], and by a stream of software programs to lose weight, improve nutrition, stop smoking, quit drinking, enhance memory, cure insomnia, end nail-biting, alleviate depression, prevent headaches, raise energy, and induce self-hypnosis, laymen are increasinely turning to the computer for expertise on matters medical.[5] Computers will show laymen how their lifespans would change if they did, or did not, exercise, smoke and so forth. Because these estimations are relatively complex, laymen will acquire these data much easier from a computer than from a book. All this, and lots more, information is going to be provided via computer in a physician's office, on-line via telephone or by the patient's own software. Beside the potentially enormous demand for health information, there could also be an even greater demand for programs which monitor illness (e.g. cardiac arrythmias) and advise on treatment. (Regrettably, these programs, especially those that can substantially affect health and disease, are not being evaluated, no less approved, by agencies in the United States, such as the Food and Drug Administration.)

Yet the post-physician era may come, less as a clinical option, and more as an economic necessity. As medical costs skyrocket, this automated self-help medical market may soon skyrocket, thereby forcing the public to look seriously at a medic-computer model. Because physician-centered and health-team models are becoming outrageously expensive, alternatives such as a medic-computer model may be resorted to out of financial desperation. The causes for escalating health-care costs are many, and a medic-computer model will not solve them all. Nevertheless, this model could greatly lower health-care costs by increasing preventive health measures, by decreasing unnecessary medical services, by reducing the physician's monopoly over health care delivery, and by introducing cost-effective incentives throughout the entire medical care system.

---

3 Maxmen, JS (1985) *The New Psychiatry: What Modern Psychiatrists Think About Their Patients, Theories, Diagnoses, Drugs, Psychotherapies, Power, Training, Family, and Private Lives*. Morrow: NY

4 Kleinfield, NR (1984) *Flood of Health Kits Widens Home Tests for Early Symptoms*. New York Times, October 1, p. Al & D4

5 A Diet and Exercise Program. Update: *Computers in Medicine*, 2(3):61, 1984; Lewis, PH (1985) Escapist Software. New York Times, p. D4

In reconsidering the post-physician era, I find the major questions are no longer technological, but matters of economics (as just mentioned) and intellect. To illustrate what I mean by "intellect", about four times a year somebody telephones me to ask: "This medical clinic has given me $300 000 to install a computer system. How can I establish the post-physician era you wrote about?" Everytime I respond with, "What do you want this system to accomplish?", my caller will admit this question never occurred to him. (A $300 000 oversight!) So intent on *having* a computer system – any computer system – its *purpose* is never considered. Computers should not be used merely because they exist, nor should a post-physician era emerge simply because it can.

Finally, in reconsidering *The Post-Physician Era*, I believe the greatest lesson of a medic-computer model is not whether it may occur, but whether the idea highlights what humans do better and worse than computers, how people can live in harmony with these machines and how we can best gain from them without our brains ossifying in the process.

10. Projecting Welfare Trends from the Past to the Future: The Example of Sweden

Mårten Lagergren

Background

In 1978 the Swedish Secretariat for Future Studies, a governmental advisory board on long-term issues of broad societal significance, began its project "Care in Society". The final project report was published in Swedish in May 1982, and an English version "Time to Care" followed in February 1984. The original purpose of the "Care in Society" project was to study how conditions in society affect the needs for care in different forms and how these needs are met, informally or through formal institutions. More broadly, the study came to be a general assessment of the welfare state and its growing problems.

The selection of the area as an object of a futures study was chiefly motivated by two observations:

1. The rapidly increasing costs for providing organized care and welfare to all citizens in need on an equal basis and the ensuing increase of the taxation level
2. The growing concern about the development of mutual care in the social networks and the growing dependency on the formal systems

Scope of the Project

The project "Care in Society" encompassed all forms of public or private organized care services (the health services, the care services for children, elderly, handicapped, etc.) as well as the mutual care in everyday life and the social welfare system (social benefits, pensions systems, etc.). The reason for including all these forms of care and welfare into one context was the great interdependence that exists between them. In many important respects they seem to act as interconnected vessels; e.g. when mutual informal care is not functioning, the pressure on the formal organized care services is increased and vice versa. Sometimes also welfare grants can be seen as a substitute for care. And all forms of publicly financed care and welfare make demands on the taxpayer.

Great emphasis was to be put on the connection between the needs of care and the conditions of society. The time perspective of the study was set at around 25 years with due consideration to the modifications that would be appropriate for different sub-problems.

Organizational Context

The study was initiated by the Secretariat for Futures Studies in 1977. The body responsible for the choice of projects and the general direction of the project work was at that time an executive committee composed of representatives of all parties in the parliament. The secretariat recruited a project group of four people for the project with the approval of the executive committee. A special ministerial reference group was also set up for the project. In 1980 the secretariat, which hitherto had had the status of a commission, was re-organized as a permanent unit attached to the Swedish Council for Planning and Coordination of Research. The executive committee was then replaced by a small delegation from the board of that agency, and the ministerial reference group was dismantled.

The project groups of the Secretariat for Futures Studies enjoy a very special freedom when it comes to choosing the ways of working and presenting their findings. After the executive committee has approved the selection of the project group and the general guidelines for its work, the group was left to decide on its own how to tackle the problems. The projects of the secretariat do not report officially to the government, but present their findings directly to the public. The executive committee (or, after 1980, the delegation) takes no responsibility for the conclusions – in fact, as was once the case, they might even go out in public and criticize a study report!

The Project Group

In composing the project group an effort was made to balance different demands: knowledge, analytic vs humanistic capability, equal representation of sexes. The result was the choice of a male systems analyst and health services planner as project director and a male urban planner, a female teacher in nursing and a female sociologist as team members.

Because of the very large and complex project area, it was felt necessary to support the project group with a group of special advisors. The six persons that were selected to that group all had broad knowledge and long experience from different fields within the problem area. The group included three medical doctors, two social workers and one journalist.

The main part of the project work was organized in the form of sub-studies, ten in all. For these sub-studies special experts were recruited as researchers, responsible for the sub-study, or as advisors. In all almost 100 persons have been involved in the study to some extent – the vast majority of these informally and with no special payment.

This involvement of different outside people in the project also served to increase the contact surface with all the different central and local government agencies, unions and university departments that are connected to the field. Apart from that, the project group also took formal contact with all the most important agencies, etc. at the start of the project, informed about its purpose and discussed with them the most important problems in their respective areas of responsibility.

Methodology

The purpose of the "Care in Society" project is perhaps best captured in the phrase that was used as title of the foregoing report under the auspices of the secretariat: "To choose a future". This means that the study was not limited to the role of a long-term prognosis. It was also designed to produce alternatives for choice. Three types of methodological problems then present themselves:

1. How to collect the information and knowledge that is needed in order to identify problems and trends
2. How to process that information in order to arrive at conclusions concerning the future of these trends, their effect and mutual influence and the consequences of alternative policies
3. How to deal with differences in values and political preferences in a parliamentary context

The first problem was handled by extensive reading and by connecting to the study group in different ways a lot of experts from different fields – most importantly perhaps through the device of sub-studies. It was agreed that the project should mainly pre-occupy itself with major, profound problems and avoid being swamped by details that could more appropriately be handled in other studies with a more restricted scope. Instead, the study was concentrated on three main features common to the whole problem area:

1. The concept of a person – values and attitudes towards our fellow man in society, mutual care and the care services
2. The professionalization of care
3. The problems of recruiting and financing the growing care services sector

From these areas other important problems were derived, such as: the organization of care services, the development of social networks, possible ways of de-professionalising care, and the employment problems of post-industrial society.

The mentioned problem areas were all treated in the form of sub-studies with special experts employed, as described above. Apart from that, special sub-studies were also devoted to the problems of children, the elderly, and the socially rejected and to the health threats of the chemical environment.

The main methodological philosophy behind the study might be labelled pluralism. Within the context of the different sub-studies, a number of various methodological approaches were used: quantitative sociological analysis, trend extrapolation, econometric modelling, hermeneutical methods. No attempt was made to unify this into a single approach. The econometric model, however, served as a general economic framework for the scenario that was presented in the final report. In this way consistency was achieved between conclusions and proposals in different sub-areas.

This model was also our main tool when it came to the treatment of uncertain factors. Extensive sensitivity analysis was performed for all significant economic parameters – production and productivity growth rate in private enterprise, labour force, wage level, immigration, working hours, treatment charges, etc. At least 500 different combinations of these parameters were analyzed.

The question of values is of course of utmost importance in a study of this kind. The problems that are treated are obviously of a political nature. On the other hand, the project had no affiliation to any special political party or interest group, and it was essential to stay away from any such connection. Instead, it was necessary to establish some kind of common ground and to develop and evaluate proposals from that base-point. This common ground was identified as the basic goals underlying the formation of the modern welfare state: full employment, social security and equal access to care regardless of income and location, and equality between the sexes.

The basic values were explicitly stated as starting points in the final report. The analysis then took the form of describing the problems involved in maintaining these goals in the future and the ways in which these problems could be mastered.

In this way it was assured that the basic values underlying the study were shared – at least in principle – by a majority of our clients, the Swedish people. This is not to say, however, that all values that entered into the study could be assumed to be generally accepted. Obviously, hundreds of decisions were made in the course of the study according to the values of the project group or its individual members. This seems unavoidable, but the analysis might still be useful to a reader with a different value system if he can incorporate his own values into the analysis and adjust assumptions and solutions accordingly. This should always be possible, in theory at least, if the analysis is presented in a scientific way with explicit assumptions upon which logical conclusions are then implemented step by step.

Output of Study and Implementation

The Main Message

The conclusions of the "Care in Society" project might perhaps best be summarized in the phrase "it can't be done". By that we mean that it does not seem possible to preserve the goals of the (Swedish) welfare state without seriously rethinking about the means that are used to achieve these goals.

We cannot continue to leave the care problems to the care professionals to be solved according to their preferences in an ever-swelling care services system. The problems of unemployment and taxation rates, that are connected to the gradual transition towards post-industrial society, also demand that a new approach be used.

Three main principles are put forward by the study:
1. Solve the care problems nearer to their source
2. Take more of the care services into our own hands
3. Increase civic control over professional care

Solving care problems nearer to their source means among other things that more emphasis must be put on health promotion and disease prevention. The second principle implies a re-valuation of non-professional care. More favourable conditions must be created for mutual care in the social networks. Voluntary care must be given a higher interest and value, and it might even be necessary to introduce a conscription system for care and other social services. Increased civic control can be achieved by decentralization of the care services system, introducing, e.g., co-operative forms of care. Medical-technological development necessitates improved procedures of prioritation. Increased lay control must also enter the relationship between caretaker and receiver of care.

Forms for Presentation and Dissemination of Results

The main message as described in the preceding paragraph evolved gradually during the later phase of the study. It was not fully developed until the presentation of the final report.

Before that, however, as mentioned above, a series of subsidiary reports were published dealing with different sub-areas and aspects of the total problem. The secretariat has created a subscription system to which a few thousand subscribers are joined – institutions and individuals. All subsidiary reports were distributed to these subscribers. This written presentation has been the most important channel to the general public. The books are also used extensively in schools for training of care services personnel of different categories. This emphasis on written reports does not mean, however, that oral presentation has been disregarded. On the contrary, the project team has been very active in presenting the analysis and conclusions of the study at conferences and courses of different kinds. This activity is still going on more than 3 years after the project has been completed!

Because of the special status of the secretariat, no formal presentation has been made to top decision-makers. Informally, however, the study has been presented to the health minister and the undersecretary of state for health and social affairs at a number of occasions.

Another way of disseminating the results of the study and starting a debate is through the mass media. Presentations have been made on television, radio and newspapers several times, mainly in connection with the publishing of reports.

These meetings with decision-makers and the public in the course of the study did constitute an important feedback – especially in the beginning of the project. The necessity of formulating ideas and conclusions in a closed form at these occasions also served to develop our thinking and to stimulate the internal discussions in the project group.

Assessment of the Impact of the Study

The impact of a study must always be assessed according to its purpose. "Care in Society" is a futures study and its impact must be evaluated as such. Four main purposes have been identified by the secretariat for its projects:

1. To evaluate long-term consequences of different policy options
2. To perform cross-sectional analysis of important societal problems
3. To stimulate the general debate concerning the future
4. To identify gaps of knowledge and needs for further research in different fields

All but the last of these four purposes seem to have been achieved fairly well by the "Care in Society" project. The last one is difficult because in such a very broad project so many gaps of knowledge are identified that it could suffice to write a programme for a large research institution for decades. Also many of the crucial problems are perhaps not researchable. Still, it would seem worthwhile to try to summarize more important problems for future research. However, this has not been done yet due to lack of resources.

As to the three other purposes, these are of course not ends in themselves. The ultimate purpose must be seen as improved decision-making and a more favourable development of society than would have occurred otherwise. Whether this will be achieved is, of course, impossible to say at this stage. Only the future can tell what influence, if any, the study will have on the development of Swedish society.

Many of the ideas proposed by the study have been received favourably by the public and the political decision-makers. The general development of the care services systems also follows the main course outlined by the study: emphasis on prevention, de-institutionalization, emphasis on primary care, decentralization, increased rights for patients, etc. However, to most of these ideas we cannot claim originality. Our task was rather to put a lot of different ideas into a common framework.

One proposition of entirely our own making – a conscription system for care – has created a lot of interest and attention to our study, at home and abroad, but has generally not attracted much support. This we did expect since the proposition obviously is a very long-term one and presupposes important changes in values and attitudes.

An interesting channel for implementation of the recommendations of the study is the new large project that has been launched by the Secretariat for Futures Studies. This project, "Municipalities and the Futures", involves eight municipalities in Sweden, which will each develop a separate, politically based, action-oriented study concerning the future of the municipality as territory and political-administrative unit. In this study, care and welfare constitute an important part, and the ideas of the "Care in Society" study are seen as starting points for local development and concrete political action.

Another aspect of the impact of the study is the lessons learned regarding methodological problems. Since, according to our knowledge, there exists no previous study of this scope (futures studies in this field have generally been confined to the health services themselves, without the societal context), the approach we have used might be of general interest. We feel that the pluralistic methodology described above has served its purpose well. It would not have been possible to treat a subject as large and varied as this one with one single approach. However, it is doubtful whether we would have been able to arrive at our conclusions without the aid of the formal computer model, since consistency is very hard to achieve without a quantitative basis.

In retrospect, the crucial problem of the study seems to have been the treatment of values and value changes. During the course of the project, important changes in attitudes occurred, or became felt, in Swedish society. The force behind this change is no doubt the economic development. It seems that an increasing number of people are not willing to take upon themselves the burden associated with continued solidarity with the weak groups of society. This development of course is an international one, not restricted to our country. The question then is whether the study should try to foresee such value changes or stick to the original value system. As described above, we have chosen the second alternative. Another possible way of course is to develop two or more alternatives. This approach was chosen in some of the sub-studies but not in the final report, since we did not find it meaningful to present a solution which we could not sympathize with. Others with different values could present such a solution much better – perhaps using facts from our analysis.

The future verdict on the "Care in Society" project is hard to predict. We believe we have succeeded fairly well in creating an overview of a complex field and thereby contributed to the understanding of the processes that are shaping the future. Undoubtedly, however, we have been prisoners of the present. Our approach and findings will be judged very typical of the thinking of the age we were working in. The future will always be different.

11. Economics, Politics and Health: The Challenge of Future Trends (A Think-Piece)

Manfred A. Max-Neef*

This think-piece is intended simply as an economist's critical reflexion, the purpose of which is to point out questions and problems for which no adequate answers are being provided by the traditional political, health and economic disciplines.

The central argument is that the new social afflictions are increasingly revealing themselves, not as specific problems, but rather as holistic problematiques that can no longer be tackled through the application of conventional policies and methodologies inspired by reductionist disciplines.

1. Just as the medical problem represented by a person's illness transcends the strict medical field when it turns into an epidemic disease, our challenge today consists not so much of confronting problems, but of confronting the tremendous magnitude of the problems.
2. The question of magnitude, more than anything else, is what determines the transformation of problems with clear disciplinary contours, into problematiques that give origin to complex transdisciplinary fields.
3. It was in the midst of the French Revolution's terror that the Marquis of Sade exclaimed: "There no longer exists any beautiful individual death!" In the midst of a present reality overwhelming us, we can exclaim in an analogous manner: "All the beautiful particular problems we are being deprived of them!"

Politics, economics and health have converged towards a crossroads. This means that health is clearly becoming a function of politics and economics. In other words, we find a growing amount of cases where bad health is the product of bad politics, and of bad economics, or of both.

We can, for instance, rightfully say that if economic policies, devised by economists, *totally* affect (as they do) *the whole* of a society, economists can no longer claim that they are only concerned with economic problems. Such a claim is highly unethical, since it implies accepting accountability for the action, but not for the consequences of the action.

We are in a mess. Things are pretty bad, and they will get worse, unless we devote much more energy and imagination to the construction of coherent and meaningful

---

* Manfred A. Max-Neef is a Chilean Economist, Founder and Managing Director of the Development Alternatives Centre – CEPAUR. For his practical and theoretical contributions to a New Economics, he was awarded the Alternative Nobel Prize in 1983

transdisciplinarities. We are in a time of far-reaching transition, which means that paradigm shifts are not only necessary, but inevitable. In the face of such a historical inevitability, procrastination (paraphrasing Fouché) is not only a crime, it is a mistake!

A Postulate and Some Propositions

Development is about people, and not about objects. This is the basic postulate of a "New Economics" and "Another Development".

The acceptance of this postulate – whether on intuitive, ethical or rational grounds – leads to the following fundamental question: "How can it be determined whether one development process is better than another?" In the traditional paradigm we have indicators such as the gross national product (GNP), which is, in a way, an indicator about the quantitative growth of objects. Now we need an indicator about the qualitative growth of people. What should that be? Let us answer the question thus: That development process will be best, which allows people's quality of life to improve the most. The next question follows: What determines people's quality of life? Quality of life will depend on the possibilities people have to adequately satisfy their fundamental human needs. The third question arises: What are those fundamental human needs, and/or who decides what they are? Some disquisitions follow before answering the question.

It is traditionally believed that human needs tend to be infinite, that they change all the time, that they are different in each culture or environment, and that they are different in each historical period. It is here suggested that such assumptions are inaccurate, since they are the product of a conceptual shortcoming.

A prevalent shortcoming in the existing literature and discussions about human needs is that the fundamental difference between *needs* and *satisfiers* is either not made explicit or is overlooked altogether. A clear distinction between both concepts is necessary, as shall be shown later, for epistemological as well as methodological reasons.

Human needs must be understood as a system: that is, all human needs are interrelated and interact. With the sole exception of the need of subsistence, that is, of being alive, no hierarchies exist within the system. Quite on the contrary, simultaneities, complementarities and trade-offs are characteristics of the process of needs satisfaction.

Now we can answer the pending question. If we disaggregate the two broad categories of needs, that is *needs of having* and *needs of being*, we suggest the following system composed of nine fundamental human needs: permanence (or subsistence), protection, affection, understanding, participation, leisure, creation, identity and freedom.[1]

---

1 See M.A. Max-Neef, C. Mallman and R. Aguirre: *Human Synergy as the Ethical and Aesthetical Foundation of Development.* Bariloche Foundation, Argentina 1978

From such a classification (which can be further disaggregated) it follows, for example, that housing, food, clothing are not to be considered as needs, but as satisfiers of the fundamental need of permanence (or subsistence). By the same token, education (whether formal or informal), early stimulation, meditation, are satisfiers of the need of understanding. Cure, prevention and health systems in general are satisfiers of the need of protection.

No one-to-one correspondence exists between needs and satisfiers. One satisfier may simultaneously contribute to the satisfaction of several needs or, inversely, a certain need may require access to several satisfiers for its satisfaction. Even these relations are not fixed. They may vary according to time, place and circumstance. One example as illustration: When a mother breast-feeds her baby, through that act, she is simultaneously contributing to the baby's satisfaction of subsistence, affection, protection and identity. The situation is obviously different if the baby is fed in a more mechanical manner.

Having separated needs from satisfiers, two basic hypotheses may be proposed. First, fundamental human needs are finite, few and classifiable. Second, fundamental human needs (as contained in the proposed system) are the same in all cultures and all historical periods. What changes, both over time and through cultures, is the form or the means by which these needs are satisfied.

Each economic, social and political system adopts different styles for the satisfaction of the same fundamental human needs. In every system they are satisfied (or not satisfied) through the generation (or non-generation) of different types of satisfiers. We may go as far as to say that one of the aspects that define a culture is its choice of satisfiers. Whether a person belongs to a consumerist or to an ascetic society, his/her fundamental human needs are the same. What changes is his/her choice of quantity and quality of satisfiers, and/or his/her possibilities of having access to the required satisfiers. In short: What is culturally determined are not the fundamental human needs, but the satisfiers for those needs. Cultural change is, among other things, the consequence of dropping traditional satisfiers for the purpose of adopting new or different ones.

The system of fundamental human needs as described may appear as somewhat static. In order to overcome such an impression it should be added that each need can be satisfied at different and, probably, increasing levels. Furthermore, they are satisfied in three contexts: (a) intra-humanly, or in relation with oneself, (b) inter-humanly, or in relation with the social group, and (c) extra-humanly, or in relation with the environment. Both the levels and the contexts, in terms of quality and intensity, will depend on time, place and circumstance.

The proposed system allows for a re-interpretation of the concept of poverty. The traditional concept of poverty is limited and restricted, since it exclusively refers to the predicaments of people who may be classified below a certain income threshold. The concept is strictly economistic. It is here suggested that we should speak not of poverty, but of poverties. In fact, any fundamental human need that is not adequately satisfied, reveals a human poverty. Some examples are: poverty of subsistence (due to insufficient income, food, shelter, etc.), of protection (due to bad health systems, violence, arms race, etc.), of affection (due to authoritarianism, oppression, exploitative relations with the natural environment, etc.), of understanding (due to bad quality of education), of participation (due to marginalization and discrimination of women, children and minorities), of identity (due to imposition of alien values upon local and regional cultures, forced migration, political exile, etc.). But poverties are not only poverties. Much more than that, *each poverty generates pathologies*. And this is the crux of our discourse.

Economics and Pathologies

The great majority of economic analysts would agree that generalized rising unemployment and Third World international indebtedness rank as the two most important economic problems of today's world. Although unemployment is a problem that has always existed in the industrial civilization to a greater or lesser degree, everything seems to indicate that now we are facing a new type of unemployment that is here to stay, because it has become a structural component of the world economic system as we know it.

It is known that a person suffering from extended unemployment goes through an emotional "roller coaster experience" which involves at least four phases: (a) shock, (b) optimism, (c) pessimism, (d) fatalism; the last phase representing the transition from stagnation to frustration, and from there to a final state of apathy, where the person reaches his/her lowest level of self-esteem. As pointed out in a Canadian report about the subject: "Losing one's job can instigate a slow and agonizing process of dying."[2] It is quite evident that extended unemployment will totally upset a person's fundamental needs system. Due to problems of subsistence, the person will feel increasingly unprotected, family crises and guilt feelings may destroy affections; lack of participation will give way to feelings of isolation and marginalization, and declining self-esteem may very well generate identity crises.

Extended unemployment generates pathologies. But, given the present circumstances of generalized economic crises, we must no longer think of pathologies as affecting individuals. We must necessarily recognize the existence of *collective pathologies of frustration*, for which we know no adequate forms of treatment.

Although it is economic processes that generate unemployment, once the latter has reached critical magnitudes, both in quantity and duration, there is no economic treatment capable of solving the problematique into which the original problem has been transformed. As a problematique it belongs to a transdisciplinarity that still remains to be understood and constructed. This, in terms of a programme for the future, represents challenge number one. As far as tendencies are concerned, these collective pathologies will increase.

---

2 S. Kirsh: *Unemployment: Its Impact on Body and Soul*. Canadian Mental Health Association, Canada 1983

International Third World indebtedness will account for other types of collective pathologies. In order to keep the international banking system corpulent and healthy, the populations in a lot of countries will have to go sick and feeble.

In early 1985 the Chairman of the British Conservative Party pointed out: "America is importing the savings of the rest of the world, and exporting the inflation. This is a very serious matter."[3] The case is that, due to an overvalued American dollar and in addition to exorbitant interest rates, the debtor nations will have to go through every pain in order to maximize their export earnings. This will inevitably occur at the expense of irreversible resources depletion, more famines and growing structural (not cyclical) impoverishment. To determine which will be the collective pathologies emerging in the poorer nations as a consequence of this aberration is challenge number two.

Only two examples have been given here. However, there are many other economic processes which, when conceived and designed in a technocratic manner and in a reductionist perspective, can generate collective pathologies. Each economist, especially those with influence over decision makers, should exercise the necessary self-criticisms in order to recognize them and anticipate their detection. This implies, of course, the willingness to adjust to a principle which is almost always forgotten: *the purpose of the economy is to serve the people, and not the other way round.*

Politics and Pathologies

Persecutions due to political, religious and other forms of intolerance are as old as humanity. However, the "achievement" of our times is the tendency of the principal political leadership of orienting their actions to such incredibly schizophrenic generalizations about "the enemy" that we are heading straight towards omnicide, that is, the killing of us all.[4] Such political schizophrenia is not only to be found at the level of global confrontations between the big powers; it also has its counterparts (mirror images) at many national levels. They are all accountable for the sprouting of many *collective pathologies of fear*.

It is here suggested that at least four categories of collective pathologies of fear should be recognized, according to their origin: (a) semantic confusion, (b) violence, (c) isolation, exile, marginalization, and (d) frustration of life projects. There are surely others, but these should suffice as examples.

The discourses of power are full of euphemisms. Words no longer fit with facts. Annihilators are called nuclear arms, as if they were simply a more powerful version

---

3 *The Guardian*, 16 February 1985

4 See the brilliant article by H. Alfvén: Annihilators and Omnicide. *Development Dialogue* 1-2, 1984 (Uppsala, Sweden)

of conventional arms.[5] We call "free world", a world full with examples of the most obscene inequities and violations of human rights. We find Democratic Republics (or People's Republics) where people must simply comply obediently with the dictums of an "almighty state". Peaceful protest marchers are severely punished and imprisoned for public disorder and subversion, while state terrorism goes as law and order. Examples could fill many pages. The case is that people cease to understand and, as a consequence, they either turn into cynics or melt into the impotent, perplexed and alienated masses.

Violence directly upsets the need of protection and security, thus giving way to intensive anxiety. Isolation, marginalization and political exile destroy a person's identity and bring about family disruptions with destroyed affections and guilt feelings often accompanied with fantasies or actual attempts at self-annihilation. Frustration of life projects by political intolerance destroys the creative capacity of people, leading them slowly from active resentment into apathy and loss of self-esteem.

Efforts to recognize and evaluate the collective pathologies, that may arise within each different socio-political system as a consequence of inhibiting the satisfaction of needs such as understanding, protection, identity, affection, creativity and freedom, is challenge number three.

Final Comments

What has been suggested in this think-piece is that:

1. Any fundamental human need not adequately satisfied generates a pathology
2. Up to the present we have developed treatments for individual, or small group, pathologies
3. Today we are faced with a dramatically increasing amount of collective pathologies for which we have devised no treatments
4. The understanding of these collective pathologies requires the prior construction of transdisciplinarities

The possibilities of bringing about a dialogue between economic, political and health disciplines that may really generate the needed transdisciplinarities is challenge number four.

Collective pathologies will grow in the near future, as well as in the long term, if we continue with traditional and orthodox approaches. It is really nonsense to individually "cure" a person, and then throw him/her back into a sick environment.

Each discipline, while becoming increasingly reductionist and technocratic, has given way to its own dehumanization. To humanize ourselves again from within our own disciplines, is the great final challenge. Only such an effort can set the

---

5 Ibid.

foundations for fruitful transdisciplinarities that may truly contribute to the solution of the real problematiques affecting our world today.

If we don't live up to our task, we will all be accomplices in the generation of sick societies. And one should not forget that if "in the land of the blind the one-eyed is king", then in sick societies it is the necrophiliacs who become the holders of power.